# Redface

# Redface

*How I Learnt to Live with Social Anxiety*

Russell Norris

First published by Canbury Press 2021
This edition published 2021

Canbury Press
Kingston upon Thames, Surrey, United Kingdom
www.canburypress.com

Printed and bound in Great Britain
Typeset by Canbury Press
Cover: Alice Marwick

This is a work of non-fiction

FSC

Printed on Forest Stewardship Council-certified paper

ISBN
Paperback: 9781912454501
Ebook: 9781912454518

*For D, Z and J.*

*You are the blessing.*

# CONTENTS

# 1. Closed doors

I'm hovering just in front of a closed door. It's in the office building where I work. I can see through the window of the door into the room beyond it. I'm listening carefully for approaching voices. As soon as another person comes into view, I'll have to make a snap decision: commit and go through that door or abort and quickly walk away from it, surreptitiously double back at some point, then try to hold my nerve for a second attempt. I've been doing this in secret for my entire career and if I could calculate exactly how much time I've lost in this state of limbo, all the seconds, minutes and hours spent holding back in hallways or pacing back and forth just behind closed doors, it might add up to a lifetime. And a waste of one.

Because there's nothing out of the ordinary on the other side of those doors. Just the usual setup of any modern workplace. Open plan desks, meeting rooms, breakout sofas, whiteboards, water coolers, tea and coffee points – spaces designed to help people work together. But people is the key word. On the other side of every door there will be people. People I know. People who know me. People I'm about to meet. People who've yet to meet me. I'm going through each door to be among other people, all day. And once I'm on the other side there's no turning back. I'll attend a meeting. A briefing. A brainstorm. I'll review some work. I'll find someone I need to speak to or I'll run into someone and they'll stop me for some small talk. I'll start to feel like I'm walking in the glare of a giant magnifying glass, growing hotter and hotter like a beam of sunshine intensifying through a lens. And if I'm not sufficiently prepared for it all, I'll start to feel something quiver and give way inside. And I'll know that if I don't escape to the other side of the door again, to the relative safety of my desk, I'll fall apart in front of everyone.

For just about as long as I can remember, I've had Social Anxiety. Not the shyness or self-consciousness everyone feels at one time or another in their lives. Not the nerves you might get before taking a driving test or going on a first date. Not the butterflies that start fluttering in your stomach before you stand up and give a speech. What lives deep inside me is an inexhaustible phobia of *any* social interaction. It creeps across all situations and all people, from the ordinarily stressful stuff like giving a presentation or having a job interview, to everyday things like buying groceries or speaking to a stranger on the phone. Presentations and interviews are nervous moments for most people: they put you at the centre of attention, while other people evaluate your performance. But the man working the checkout in Sainsbury's? The woman taking my pizza order over the phone? Are they putting me in the spotlight, assessing my social performance? No, they're not. But I feel anxious dealing with them nonetheless. Big events, small events, everything in between: they all distress me in ways I can't control.

Phobias like mine are driven by a primal emotion: fear. Fear is one of evolution's most basic instincts. It keeps us safe and helps us survive, but when it falls out of kilter with its stimulus, it becomes unnatural and a burden. In general, buttons do not evoke fear, nor do trees or the colour yellow. But some people are scared witless by buttons (*Koumpounophobia*), trees (*Hylophobia*), or anything yellow (*Xanthophobia*). I have a close friend who's afraid of mayonnaise (a genuine phobia that is unnamed, as far as I can tell). These very specific fears sound silly to most people. It's hard to understand how mundane things could ever fill a person with dread. The people who are afraid of these things can't make sense of it either. They know buttons, trees, bananas, or mayonnaise are totally harmless and their response is irrational. That makes their feelings even more distressing.

Likewise, I know that daily contact with other human beings does not pose a threat to me. It can't hurt me physically and it's not meant to hurt me mentally. Yet it does. And I know I'm not the only one. Social Anxiety Disorder (SAD) is formally classed as a mental disorder, which affects millions of people worldwide – and up to 10% of the UK population. It can manifest itself in many ways. Symptoms often surface as secondary phobias, ranging from a fear of eating or writing in front of others to a fear of being watched in a public bathroom. For me, social anxiety plays out on my skin.

Although I'm half American with 1/28th Native American blood, I was born and raised in the UK and I have typically pale English skin. It's sensitive skin. If I scratch an itch, the spot I've touched turns bright red for the next few minutes. I sunburn faster than anyone else I know. When I'm hot, my skin goes red. When I'm cold, my skin goes red. When I'm completely at rest in a room with the perfect temperature, my skin still glows faintly red. It's my default colouring, deepening to a fiery crimson when I blush. And blushing is something that happens to me absurdly often. A blush is an uncomfortable experience and usually triggered by social error. It happens when we make a mistake or an interpersonal faux pas. I don't just go red when I'm embarrassed. I can blush at any time, in any place – frequently during mundane events like talking to friends, buying something in a shop, asking someone for directions or simply making eye contact with another human being.

When the blush itself starts becoming the social error, when you blush in circumstances that wouldn't usually trigger a blush, it becomes a source of fear. This fear is called *Erythrophobia*. Its symptom is called *Idiopathic Craniofacial Erythema*, which means uncontrollable and unprovoked facial blushing. They are the evil twins who constantly embarrass me. When I blush it's involuntary and I have no control over it. Because I have no control over it, I fear it happening. And because I fear it happening, it happens more. It's a feedback loop that reinforces itself over and over, until the blushing spills out into the primary phobia of social anxiety. What makes me blush? The presence of people. What will stop the blushing? The absence of people. Will there ever be a world without people? No. Will I try to create that world for myself? Yes. I have to. I will withdraw and avoid human contact whenever I can.

When I was younger, when my social anxiety was burning at its brightest, that's how I used to think. Round and round the irrational cycle would go, pulling me deeper into myself, into my own bubble, where I wouldn't have to deal with an endless succession of people and the constant threat of blushing. All through my teens and most of my twenties, social anxiety drove everything I did. It decided where I went, who I met, who I became friends with (and more often who I didn't become friends with). It determined my personality, my habits, my worldview. It dictated my every move in an elaborate and strategic scheme, designed to avoid people at all costs.

Because what sits at the very core of social anxiety is avoidance. It's a force that grips your shoulders and steers you away from anything that might trigger your distress. Social Anxiety Disorder is often described as 'the illness of missed opportunities' because it diverts your energy into the sidelines, into a life that runs parallel to the mainstream. It's almost like spending a life in hiding. In the short term, SAD makes you miss parties, skip nights out, avoid group meals. It makes you avoid new faces. Avoid old friends. It even makes you avoid your own family. In the long term, if avoidant behaviour grows unchecked — feeding on itself again and again — it can devastate a person. You might miss out on a fulfilling career or a meaningful relationship; you might not meet the right partner and have children.

Which all sounds incredibly bleak, doesn't it? It certainly felt bleak to me through my youth. I didn't know what social anxiety was until I reached my mid twenties. And that's the bleakest part of all: so many people with Social Anxiety Disorder don't even know it has a name. They struggle through life with it feeling quietly cursed, believing there's something fundamentally wrong with them.

With the bad, though, can come the good. Distressing as it was when I was a kid, social anxiety helped my education. Out of a dread of people grew a love of books. After school, I embarked on a degree in English Literature, and, after university, a career as a writer. I wasn't very confident in a room, but I was on a page. So I became a junior copywriter and, many years later, Head of Copy at an advertising agency. I wouldn't be here today, writing this book right now, if social anxiety hadn't made me avoid people in my younger years. It helped me find my profession and sharpen my skills. What I considered my weakness ended up becoming my strength. They say curses always contain blessings, even if you can't see them right away. So:

If you have social anxiety, this book is for you.

If you've never heard of social anxiety, this book is for you.

I've been quietly avoiding people all my life, hesitating behind a door. But I'm pushing that door wide open now. And I'm coming through it.

To talk to you.

# 2. Blushing

I can't remember when I first blushed. It's been happening to me for so long now that it's hard to pinpoint when it began. But I do remember when I didn't blush. Before I went to secondary school, all through primary school and up to the age of 11, I don't remember blushing at all. Or it wasn't something I was especially conscious of. And consciousness plays the critical role in blushing. Take it away and a blush will not exist.

When I left primary school, I was confronted by new places, new faces, new rules, a new sense of identity. My consciousness shifted from 2D into 3D. It took on a new dimension. I became more aware of other people, more aware of how they responded to each other and that how I behaved affected the things they said and did to me. Day by day, week by week, month by month, I became more aware of myself. And it didn't take long for my awareness to tip over into self-consciousness. By my early teens, when I was 12 or 13 years old, I was already blushing.

And I had no idea of the power it would come to have over my adult life. I'll have to be careful how I talk about blushing because language lets me down. It makes me own the blush: *I blushed, my blushing*. It doesn't explain how I feel. As far as I've always been concerned, a blush is something that happens to me. I am not the active 'doer'. I'm entirely passive. Much like a yawn you can't stifle or a hiccup or a sneeze: when I blush, it's entirely involuntary. But unlike other involuntary bodily actions – when your eyes blink, when your mouth salivates, when your skin itches – when your face blushes, there is no physiological benefit to be had. No clear biological purpose is being served. The function is purely social.

I started blushing as a young teenager and I still blush today as a 40-year-old man. The blushing has grown less frequent and less fierce with time but it's still very much with me, every minute of every day. A blush might seem harmless or maybe even charming to someone who rarely experiences one. But it's distressing to be a blusher and doubly so if you're male and no longer an adolescent. Because, as much as we live in an age of equality and I want to believe things like gender and age don't define who we are, our social codes and norms run deep. Unconscious bias runs the deepest.

Historically, blushing has been viewed as feminine. Something that's becoming for a woman but questionable in a man. In Thomas Hardy's 19th century novel *Far from the Madding Crowd*, the farm-hand Joseph Poorgrass is a painfully chronic blusher. When he confides to his fellow workers that blushing has made his life difficult, someone remarks: "Tis a very bad affliction for ye, Joseph...'tis very well for a woman...'tis awkward for a man.' Which is old-fashioned thinking, to be sure. But old-fashioned tropes can stay in currency. Just think of British phrases like 'the blushing bride' or 'an English rose', both used to describe a fair woman with a rosy complexion. Shakespeare himself described a reddened face as 'a maiden blush'. In ways we might not acknowledge, it's hard-coded into our society that blushing is somehow effeminate. Which is equally unfair to men and women. A blushing woman is no more comfortable with her blush than a blushing man. And yet, with a man, an extra stigma is attached. For a man amongst men, blushing feels like a bit of a weakness. It sends out the signal you're a Beta male.

Imagine the typical Hemingway man, showing smooth macho grace under pressure. Imagine Don Draper in *Mad Men* being suave, composed and unreadable. Imagine Tom Hardy in almost every role he's played: cool, strong, decisive. These are flat caricatures of manliness, no doubt, but as cultural stereotypes they've been around for centuries. You might think you aren't affected by such things — that your thoughts on gender roles and neutrality are entirely your own — but the human brain thrives on preconceived models and stereotypes. It craves them. Our gut reactions are shaped by emotions we often can't explain. Can you imagine a storyline about Tom Hardy getting a bit flustered and turning red when he's challenged to a fight? No one would ever make that film and no one would pay to watch it. It's not a movie I would want to see, even. But why is it my natural reaction to think a socially awkward Tom Hardy would be pointless viewing? It's my own unconscious bias poking through. I've been given an idea of what a leading man should be. And leading men do not blush at the slightest provocation. Men who blush involuntarily send out a message to everyone else: they have a weakness that they should've outgrown by now.

Blushing also suggests immaturity and inexperience. There's something almost virginal about it. It doesn't belong in the adult world because by the time you're an adult, you should be able to control your emotions — unlike a child who throws a temper tantrum, cries hysterically, or runs away and hides his face. Childhood is defined by lack of control. Adulthood by its steady accumulation. To have not gained control of your blushing by the time you're a grown-up, living among grown-ups... well, it almost suggests you're underdeveloped. Like a part of your emotional education went missing. As though part of you still has a lot of growing up left to do.

You might not think like this at all when you see someone blush. Research shows that a blush is often interpreted as a sign of trustworthiness. If you find it hard to conceal your true emotions, so the thinking goes, you will find it harder to deceive people. Thus you are 'more genuine.' On the other hand, if you're someone who seldom blushes, it's seen as especially attractive when you do. 'I can't even imagine how handsome that man must be blushing,' says Joan about Don Draper in *Mad Men*. It's such a rarity to see a chink in Don's armour that when you finally do, it's almost thrilling.

But for those on the other side of the fence, for the adults who are prone to blushing, they never see things this way. They over-think it. They wonder if other people think they're not being a 'real' man. Or if they're just being a 'typical' woman. They spend time worrying that others find them childish or submissive, weak or unprofessional, overly sensitive or difficult. Sometimes it's perfectly natural to blush. Saying something inappropriate by accident, for example. Or being teased by someone you fancy. The blush response serves a clear social purpose and it's the equivalent of letting your guard down. It's a unique signal that you are human and your human nature sometimes gets the better of you. But for some people, myself included, two factors combine to make blushing uncommonly frequent: an introverted character and an over-active sympathetic nervous system.

Much has been written about introversion in recent years. Susan Cain sparked a new cultural movement with her inspirational book *Quiet: The Power of Introverts in a World That Can't Stop Talking*. Her exploration – exoneration – of the introverted mindset can't be bettered. She made it OK to be reserved, to be quiet, to prefer your own company in what has largely become an out-there extroverted world. But at the core of her argument, she makes a very important distinction between introverted people and shy people: 'Shyness and introversion are not the same thing. Shyness is the fear of negative judgement. Introversion is a preference for quiet, less stimulating environments.'

I like to call myself an introvert, that I simply prefer less stimulating environments. It's currently cool to be an introvert. It's a trendy subject on LinkedIn and Twitter and it keeps cropping up in TED talks. So I've happily adopted the label to make my social unease more acceptable to myself. But I can't escape the nagging voice in the back of my head that says I'm just shy. The OED defines shyness as 'diffident or uneasy in company' and that describes me perfectly. Shyness lives at the less desirable end of introversion and it doesn't quite fit into any brave new world. My shyness comes from a fear of negative social judgement, as defined by Susan Cain. But it's also driven by something deeper. My shyness is fuelled by an intense awareness that I am here. Every second, I exist. And every second I feel inherently uncomfortable inside my own skin.

It's an involuntary mental and emotional state. And it's compounded by an equally involuntary physical state: an over-active sympathetic nervous system. Within the human nerve circuits is a complex called the Autonomic Nervous System. It controls your body's unconscious activities, the things that happen without your mental input like your digestion, your heart rate, your uninterrupted breathing when you're fast asleep. It splits off into three branches and one of them, the Sympathetic Nervous System, controls your 'fight-or-flight' response. Fight-or-flight is an ancient survival mechanism that jolts your body into alertness, to either engage in a fight or flee from it, so you can live to fight another day. Effectively, it releases a spurt of adrenaline and hormones into your bloodstream to snap you into defensive or offensive action. It's what helps you dodge a speeding cyclist, for example. Or instinctively catch a falling glass. Or protect your face from a punch. Or, even better, to throw the punch yourself before someone else punches you. Essentially it's a good thing. It's designed to keep you safe. But if you're hypersensitive to this kind of arousal, if your Sympathetic Nervous System responds disproportionately, this bodily function can overwhelm you to the point that it starts to creep into your mental character. You've heard of people being described as 'highly strung', 'uptight', 'wound up' or 'on edge'? These are words for someone who's never truly relaxed, someone who's always tense. These people are reacting to their Sympathetic Nervous System, which in turn is working on overtime. This is me.

My wife is always laughing because I'm so jumpy. If we're walking down the road and a siren goes off before I see the police car coming, I jump out of my skin. When a fast train flies past me on the platform each morning, blasting its horn to keep passengers well back — I jerk so violently that I almost fall onto the tracks. I've always disliked balloons because they can pop with a pistol-like bang at any given moment; and I find it stressful watching children play with them — waiting for their teeth or nails to dig into the taut, stretched rubber and set off the inevitable BANG! If I'm at the theatre and a character pulls out a gun, I instinctively put one finger into my ear to dampen the sound of the shot. I get twitchy at Christmas or on New Year's Eve when people hand out the party poppers — so many mini explosions just waiting to go off and it's impossible to predict when each one will. I can't genuinely say I enjoy fireworks, especially if I'm close-up to the action. I slip into a mild kind of fugue, dreading the next pyrotechnic boom to the point that I can't hold proper conversations.

Fireworks explode in one of my earliest memories. I'm three years old, it's Guy Fawkes Night and my parents have taken my sister and I to a fireworks display in the park. I'm bundled up in a puffy winter coat and woolly hat, holding my dad's hand tight as we walk slowly under gigantic trees full of flickering orange and yellow leaves. We join a crowd surging towards a giant bonfire, burning red in the middle of a football pitch. My dad lifts me up so I can get a better look above the heads in the crowd. I don't remember the first few explosions going off. I don't remember any actual fireworks at all. At this point my memory shifts with a flash to me wailing into my dad's shoulder while he carries me as fast as he can back to the car, his voice trying to soothe me and calm me down. We're heading back towards the main road and as we pass the entrance to the park my dad buys me a toffee apple – the first toffee apple I've ever seen – and once we're safely back inside the parked car, with the windows up and the heater on, he gives it to me. I sniff and sob and nibble dejectedly at the hard caramelised sugar while fireworks silently burst into colour far away on the other side of the windscreen.

I've never forgotten that. It feels like it was the true beginning, before the self-consciousness and before the blushing. It was the first time the external world became too much. The first sign that my senses were primed for overload.

Everything I've described so far has been based on sound. The sympathetic nerves are also in charge of typically 'nervy' reactions like sweating and shaking. If they are turned up to the max, your heart rate will increase with very little provocation. You will sweat more readily than others when you feel uncomfortable. And the capillaries in your face will dilate much more freely when your brain perceives the slightest hint of a threat: you will blush more easily.

What was once designed to give us a physical advantage now has the power to put us at a psychological disadvantage. Bring together a hypersensitive body and a shy mind and you have a uniquely human problem. You create a vortex of social anxiety.

# 3. Fast, slow and vicious

Charles Darwin was intrigued by the prospect of blushing. He devoted a whole chapter to it in *The Expression of the Emotions in Man and Animal*. As he correctly reasoned back in 1872, its cause is entirely mental – yet its effect is so immediately physical. It's the physicality and visibility of blushing that makes it such an uncomfortable experience. Darwin theorised that blushing runs in families, happens across all races and serves a common evolutionary function: it signals your regard for the opinions of others. He also touched upon the two different ways that people experience this 'most peculiar and the most human of all expressions'.

One is blushing, the other is flushing. Although I'd prefer to call them the Fast Blush and the Slow Blush.

When I'm assailed by a Fast Blush, I exhibit the classic blush response. Something happens that pricks my self-consciousness into action, the blood vessels in my face dilate and fill with blood, my whole face deepens through several shades of red and then, about 30 seconds later, the blood drains away again and my skin returns to its natural colour. It's all over in under a minute. While it lasts it's impossible to miss. Anyone who looks at me while I'm blushing will see what's happening to my face – and draw their own conclusions.

Just about anything can trigger a Fast Blush. It can be something unexpected, like someone coming over to my desk to talk to me at work or someone asking for my thoughts in a meeting. It can be something fully anticipated, like giving my order to a waiter or greeting a friend I've arranged to meet. There's no rhyme or reason to it. It's infuriatingly inconsistent. Some days I blush much less easily, much less frequently. Other days I'll feel blood rising up into my face at the slightest thing. Those are usually the days when I'm ultra-jumpy. The slightest change in my situation will fire off the blush. I find I'm more like that when I've had too much sugar or caffeine. Or when I'm hungover. My nerves stretch out taut like the skin on a snare drum. Just the slightest contact with anything else makes them skitter and snap.

I know when a Fast Blush is on its way. I get a quick tingling sensation somewhere inside my chest, just below the base of my throat. Like chemicals mixing together. This is the spark, if you will. And my face is the tinder. Right when someone (or even something) catches me off guard, I feel this hidden spark burst into life. I feel a second or two of sinking dread. That's it, here comes the blush. Then the gates open and hot blood begins to spread, rapidly and evenly, through every millimetre of my face.

And I can see exactly when the person or people I'm talking to notice the blush. Their eyes leave mine and start roaming around my face, as though they're following the path of a fast-moving insect as it crawls across my forehead, over my cheeks, down my neck. They look momentarily surprised. They might stare for a moment too long, as people naturally do when something happens out of the blue. They'll raise their eyebrows and a half-question will form on their lips. They'll visibly want to ask me why I've suddenly turned so red.

A lot of people keep this question to themselves. Instinctively, they know it's bad form to call it out. Call it empathy. Call it tact. When they ignore the fact I'm blushing and carry on talking as normal, I'm always grateful. It tells me they're on my wavelength and we can mutually push the blush to one side and just get on with things.

I remember meeting a man at a party once, a complete stranger I found myself standing next to at the bar. We said hello, introduced ourselves and did what you normally do when you first meet a new acquaintance – we both extended our arms to shake hands. Except this man had no hand. And no forearm. His limb ended abruptly at the elbow, where three shrivelled fingers hung in a limp bunch. I froze with my arm poised in mid-air. It was quite possibly the very last thing I'd been expecting.

It's amazing how fast the human brain can process thought. Without saying these words to myself or stopping to think them through, my brain instantly flew down a well-trodden path of reasoning:

*Imagine how often this guy meets a new person who tries to shake his hand. Imagine how tiresome it must be, every single time, to watch that person freeze or recoil when they notice his disfigurement. To know in advance, every single time, that it's going to play out in exactly the same way. To come to expect it, then hate it, then fear it. To have it slowly chip away at you and your faith in other people. Over the months, the years and the decades: this simple act of friendliness that so quickly becomes unkind.*

This took a split second. Long enough for me to recover my momentum and keep reaching out to grab the man's stump. I gripped it tightly in my palm and shook his arm up and down. I launched straight back into our conversation as though nothing out of the ordinary had happened. And being a blusher helped me do it. Because people who blush are familiar with this predicament.

Every time the blood rushes into their face, they know that for every person who politely ignores it there'll be another person who'll doggedly zero in on it. They'll ask the age-old question that makes all blushers squirm. *Why have you gone so red?*

There are lots of variations on this theme. There's the point-blank observation. *You've turned so red!*

There's the rhetorical question. *Do you know how red you've gone?* (Of course I do. How could I be unaware of it? When I blush, I'm aware of little else.)

There's the goading challenge. *Could you possibly get any redder?*

There's the wider appeal for humiliation. *Hey, look how red he's gone!* This last one is probably the worst, rooted as it is in a cruel instinct to gouge the wound. Once a cocky colleague announced to a roomful of about 30 people: *Look how red that face is. Do you think Russell has an actual medical problem?*

When people do draw attention to my blushing, much rarer these days but a daily (almost hourly) event in my schooldays, a Fast Blush can switch on the afterburners and redouble itself. A second blush rises up underneath the first, making it twice as powerful, and last twice as long.

When I was younger, I used to fantasise about what it would be like to have darker skin. The blood would be less visible in my face, I wouldn't have to worry about constantly going red, I'd be more confident and talkative and sociable, I'd have more friends, I'd meet more girls, I'd be more present and outgoing in everything I did. In short I'd be a different person.

My wife is British-Indian, born and raised in London by Punjabi parents who moved to Britain in the 1970s. I was naturally attracted to her dark hair, brown eyes and bronze skin. Her personality and character too; but that came later. They say it takes just one second to know if you're physically attracted to someone. It's coded into your neural networks, where your brain makes instant decisions for you. Attractive? Yes or no? Pale white skin, prone to blotchiness or blushing, gets a no from my brain. It's an involuntary reaction, much like a blush itself, and it stems from my dislike of my own appearance. It's a prejudice against anyone like me.

The second kind of blush is the Slow Blush. It's arguably worse than a fast one because it takes longer to reach its peak and much longer to go away. It usually begins with a Fast Blush, though. The spark, the blood flooding the face, the knowledge that people have just seen me turn red. But if I'm in an environment I can't easily escape from, for example a group discussion, it will turn into a Slow Blush. And if I'm in a formal situation like a presentation or a serious one-on-one meeting – if it's any situation that makes me the focus of attention, in a space where I'm expected to remain present and can't slip away — if it's anything official, from a boardroom to a dinner table, I'm in trouble.

I've never witnessed the onset of a Slow Blush in the mirror and I don't need to. I can tell where the blush is making itself known by the heat in my face. It begins on the top of my cheekbones, feeling like the tips of two red-hot pokers burning through my skin. Then the fire spreads outwards across my cheeks. This is usually when I notice people looking at me differently. Their gaze lingers for slightly too long as they mentally assess the change. Then my neck begins to feel like it's having an allergic reaction. It tingles and gets irritated, like I'm wearing a roll-neck jumper made from scratchy wool. I get a sensation like prickly heat, as though I'm trapped in a shaft of intensely bright sunlight and I can't move aside to find shade. Waves of heat pulse up through the neck of my shirt so that my head feels like it's floating on a draught of hot air. If things get really bad, I'll break out in a sweat: in the obvious places like the forehead and under the armpits but also on my chest and stomach. I'll look down at my shirt and see wet patches forming. My anxiety will rise higher.

The Slow Blush is painfully slow. And once it's taken hold, it's painfully unpleasant. It's happened to me thousands of times but I don't think it will ever get easier to go through. My face and neck become mottled all over in scarlet, like someone has just thrown scalding water at my head. The blood stays there, boiling hot and pulsing all over my face in irregular patches that stand out in stark contrast to my white skin. I look like a man in distress, having some kind of physical meltdown. My mouth starts twitching, my eyes dart furtively around the room as I watch people picking up on my situation one by one. I always tell myself: *It's not that bad. You're just getting a little bit rosy. A bit hot and bothered. Don't let it become a big deal.* I try to fool myself that it's a small complication and I'll soon have it under control, in a vain attempt to slow my heartbeat and reduce the surging adrenaline.

But when the meeting or presentation ends and it becomes acceptable for me to escape the room, I head straight to the nearest toilets and lock myself inside a cubicle. Reluctantly, I glance in the mirror, just to see how bad it really got. And most of the time, it's at the worse end of bad. My face will be splattered all over in vivid red blotches. The arteries in my neck will be visibly ticking with blood. My heart sinks, as I think about what the other people in the room must have thought about me when they saw my face slowly erupt in a cacophony of red. I think about the fact that I'm over 40 now and this is still happening to me so easily. That part of my life is largely out of control — and my daily dread of it is a self-contained secret. I look at my watch, sit down on top of the toilet seat, close my eyes and try to take long, measured breaths. It will be at least 20 minutes before I can get up and leave. I can't go back now, not with my face looking like this. I hear a tap dripping in another cubicle, echoing off the cold tile walls. The toilets are utterly still and empty. And for those next 20 minutes, I feel very much on my own.

The Fast Blush, the Slow Blush. They both add up to the same thing. They're upsetting experiences I wish to avoid. So they become the driving force in a mental cycle. Compulsive eaters often describe their behaviour with self-fulfilling prophecies like: I eat because I'm unhappy, I'm unhappy because I eat. By trying to escape from their problem they end up reinforcing it. I've always wanted to avoid blushing. Hence, I've always avoided situations that might make me blush. The more I avoid these situations, the more I fear them. And the more I fear them, the more they make me blush. The cycle will happily continue forever — unless you break it. It took me years to recognise this cycle for what it was. And just how strongly it had gripped me.

It's made up of three stages: Before, During and After. These are the core ingredients of social anxiety.

# 4: Before

When I was still at school, towards the end of Sixth Form, a friend of mine decided to tell me exactly what he thought about my blushing.

'Here's the thing about you, Russ. When people are in a lesson or in assembly and someone puts their hand up to ask a question... OK, they might get self-conscious and go a bit red when they start to talk and the whole room turns around to look at them. But the thing with you, is... you put your hand up and start going red before the teacher even notices you want to say something.'

He didn't know it at the time, but what he so candidly described was the very essence of anxiety: incessant worry about something that hasn't happened yet.

And by 'something that hasn't happened yet' I don't mean hypothetical scenarios like 'what if a terrorist blows up my train tomorrow?' or 'I wonder if an asteroid will end life on Earth?'. That sort of worry is better classed as angst or ennui. I'm talking about an imminent, tangible event. Think about any situation that makes you anxious: sitting an exam, giving a speech, singing karaoke. At what point does it start to make you anxious? The day before it happens? The morning before it happens? The hour beforehand? Capture that feeling in your mind as you recall the onset of your anxiety: something is coming your way that will force you outside of your comfort zone. It fills you with a sense of foreboding, of doubt, of dread. And the simplest way to describe it is stage-fright.

Stage-fright is performance anxiety, the knowledge that you will soon be judged by the quality of your performance. Classically, it describes actors or musicians who suddenly find themselves terrified of the spotlight. It's something you'd think wouldn't bother the pros who make performances look easy on stage and screen. But it's incredibly common, from theatrical greats like Michael Gambon ('It came on a couple of years ago and now it's dangerous for me to do stage plays.') to international movie stars like Hugh Grant ('I really don't know where it suddenly came from. It would just hit me in the middle of a film... but it was devastating.')

For the rest of us the stage is anywhere you have to give a

performance that's out of the ordinary. Such moments tend to have heightened consequences. Do well in an interview and you might get the job. Impress the boss in a presentation and you might get the promotion. Wow the crowd with your speech and you'll win respect from your peers. The nerves are justified. You could even say that they're proof that you care about your latest endeavour; they stoke the fire in your belly to achieve more. People who give a knockout performance sometimes credit that extra impetus for making the difference. For others, though, nerves can become all-consuming and sabotage success.

Have you read *Lucky Jim*? It's a very funny tale about a young lecturer, breaking all the stuffy rules of higher education in 1950s Britain. In the novel, Jim the anti-hero knows he has to give an important lecture to a hall full of students and professors. He can't avoid the talk and knows he'll have to give it, but he keeps putting it to the back of his mind. It floats in and out of the story, a vague threat in the future creeping closer and closer with each passing chapter. When the day of his speech finally arrives, Jim has prepared all of his notes but he hasn't sufficiently prepared his mind. As the hour draws near, he drinks beer, then whisky to try to calm his nerves. It's a big mistake and he takes to the podium in a haze of jitters and booze – and in one of literature's most famous meltdowns, delivers a catastrophic public address that ends with him falling unconscious on-stage.

It's an exaggerated depiction of stage-fright and what it can do to an otherwise self-collected person. But there's another kind of extreme. It happens at the other end of the scale, where the everyday moments of no real importance take place. At this end of the scale, small things get magnified into big things. It's where something run-of-the-mill becomes just as terrifying as a big public speech.

'Don't worry about the future; or worry, but know that worrying is as effective as trying to solve an algebra equation by chewing bubblegum.' That was the twee but sage advice dispensed by Mary Schmich, a journalist whose manifesto for a happier life went viral back in 1997 and gave Baz Luhrmann the lyrics to his *Sunscreen Song*. Schmich was totally right: worrying is futile. It's a helpless state of panicked waiting, much what I imagine it's like for lost souls living in limbo. Worrying is inaction and it cannot solve a problem. Only action can solve a problem. If it's possible to solve something, you don't need to worry about it. If it's impossible to solve something, then equally, you don't need to worry about it.

That's a perfectly rational way to think. I wish my brain could be trained to follow that logic. But worry doesn't bow down to logic. Just like everybody else I worry about the things I can and can't change. Like everybody else, I worry about the big scary events that come along every once in a while to put me to the test. Trouble is, social anxiety makes me worry about all the trivial things too. The tiny events that happen so often there should be zero reason to worry about them at all.

When I'm working with ad agencies, I come into work every day to attend a morning *stand-up*. It's a quick team meeting lasting 15 minutes max. During a stand-up, all team members come together and stand in a circle. One by one, they tell the group what they did yesterday, what they're doing today and if anything's blocking their progress. It happens every single day. It's embedded in everyone's work routine just like having your lunch or stopping for a tea break. But every single day, just before a stand-up begins, I feel my nerves flick into life. It reminds me of a pilot light inside a gas boiler. As soon as I start thinking about the imminent stand-up, my anxiety flicks on – ready to boil up the tank at a moment's notice. It's better if I'm one of the first to speak. I share my updates before my worry builds up and let the discussion move on. But if I'm further along the circle, I get more and more anxious as the conversation slowly makes its way around to me. I start to over-analyse what I'm going to say, I imagine myself going blank and having nothing to contribute, of blushing in front of everyone. I struggle to take in what my other colleagues are saying because I'm so preoccupied by what might happen when my turn arrives.

I should add that these stand-ups pretty much always pass without a hitch. I always remember what I want to say, I never freeze or clam up or make a fool of myself in public. And yet it stays with me: a small persistent fear, making itself known every day I turn up for work.

Once every week, I used to host a team meeting for a small team of five talented writers. My responsibility was to keep the meetings regular and interesting. Most weeks, I'd prepare a theme to discuss or a video to watch. It was never a formal affair. People turned up with coffee and biscuits, ready to chat and catch up and swap their news. It was nothing but casual talk. However – and this is something you'll hear a lot of introverts or people with SAD say – I find small talk difficult to navigate. For some people, chit-chat is effortless. They can somehow fill minute after minute with free-flowing talk, never running aground on an awkward silence, always armed with their next topic to steer the conversation in a new direction. And I admire that. But I find it hard to emulate. Without prompts from other people or enough time to think my thoughts through, I often struggled to think of things to say. And so I sometimes struggled to run the meeting, relying on the buzz of other people to keep it ticking along. Each week, as I walked into the meeting room, 30 minutes suddenly felt like an age to keep a group of people talking. By the end of half an hour, I felt physically tired and a sensation of gratitude rippled through me as I left the room. I'd made it through another team meeting and it would be a whole week before I had to manage the next one.

At my old agency, I was usually asked to present to a client once a month or so. I almost preferred it when it happened at short notice, so I didn't have time to stew in my own juices. More often, though, I was given plenty of warning. Let's say a week. I'd be told to take the client through some new writing my agency had produced. Some tone of voice guidelines or maybe some new copy for an app. You'd think that some forward notice was a good thing. A week gave me time to prepare my work and compose my arguments, right? Not really. In truth, more time just gave my phobia more oxygen to breathe.

The moment the date was set for my client meeting, my stage-fright began. The future threat floated up like a black zeppelin on the horizon, a looming menace slowly drifting closer every day. I would worry about it for days in advance. It would always be at the back of my mind, making itself known with persistent murmurs. *The presentation's coming in six days. Five days. Four days. All eyes will be on me. I'd better be engaging. I'd better be convincing. The presentation's coming and there's nothing I can do about it.* By the time the big day arrived, my anxiety had blown itself out of all proportion to the task being asked of me. I was simply giving a presentation to people who wanted to hear it, but I felt like I was about to storm the beaches at Normandy. No one was holding a gun to my head. No one was asking me to jump out of an aeroplane. This was simply how business was done. Yet it routinely terrified me.

I found out some years ago that physical exercise soothes my nerves. If I go for a long run the night before I have to speak or present to a group, I feel noticeably less anxious the next day. And I definitely blush less. Exercise lowers blood pressure and consumes excess energy. For me, it burns up lots of the surplus adrenaline that always seems to be flowing through my bloodstream. And so I find myself arranging my exercise around my work diary. Got a big meeting on Friday? I'll run on Thursday night. The client's coming in first thing on Monday? Then Sunday night is run night. It's doubly helpful by suppressing my nerves and keeping me fit. It's by no means a cure, though. A run doesn't guarantee calmer nerves. There have been many times when I've expected exercise to help but it's made no real difference at all. It's further evidence of the irrational, unpredictable nature of social anxiety. Sometimes I can't always squeeze in a long run before every important work engagement. When that happens, I resort to other coping strategies (more on those later.)

Stand-ups, team meetings, client presentations are just three examples of when and how my stage-fright manifests. But it doesn't stop there: it seeps into every nook and cranny of my working day. If I see an email arrive in my inbox or a message pop up on Slack, asking me to 'go and catch up with so-and-so' or 'jump on a call with what's-her-name', my heart skips a beat. And then it sinks a little. Because then I'll have to go and find these people, to initiate a conversation in a crowded room – something I still find hard to do, no matter how well I know the people I'm about to go and see.

Frankly, it's exhausting. And because it happens all the time, people with SAD find themselves on a continual search for relief. It leads to what psychologists call 'avoidance: a maladaptive coping mechanism characterised by the effort to avoid dealing with a stressor.' In short, it's when you believe that the more you distance yourself from a problem, the less it will trouble you. It's the equivalent of sticking your head in the sand. Avoidance starts small but ends big and it's a dangerous path to go down. Avoidance quickly gets coded into your mental DNA. It's possibly the hardest habit for someone with SAD to break free from, once it's taken root.

I used to avoid a hell of a lot early in my career. I was professionally evasive and it always left me feeling disappointed. The word 'avoid' implies a choice: the option was there to do something, but you chose not to. These days I have less of a choice at work. My career has moved on and more is expected of me. So now, I have to walk towards intimidating social situations. No matter what might happen.

Let's look at what does happen, and why it's so strangely traumatic.

# 5: During

If you've ever had a panic attack, you've tasted social anxiety. Panic attacks suddenly hit you with a host of symptoms: a wildly beating heart, uncontrollable sweating, trembling muscles, physical numbness, hyperventilation. They all add up to an overwhelming feeling that something truly terrible is about to happen.

But these are symptoms. And they usually point back to something else. It could be anything from an underlying panic disorder or post traumatic stress disorder to ongoing depression or drug abuse. Panic is a definitive component of SAD because it leads to the very thing that people living with it wish to avoid: a total loss of control in public. I can't say I experience all of these symptoms every time my social anxiety runs away from me. I don't become breathless, for example. And it's never made any part of my body go numb. But the thumping heart? The sweats? The shakes? Yes, yes and yes. Plus a few other symptoms, besides.

I'm going to state the inescapable again: my anxiety is triggered by human beings. And human beings are everywhere. In work, in play, in every shade of life in between, I'm always close to people. And that means I'm always close to a new and potentially humiliating social situation.

Here's an everyday scenario that passes unremarkably for most people but routinely puts me in distress. I've always had a particular aversion to communal eating. It's not a fear of eating in public places; I'll happily eat my lunch in a crowded cafeteria or on a bench in a busy park (although I never like to be the guy who's stuffing his face with a cheeseburger on the last train home on Friday night, while the rest of the carriage glares at him in disgust). What makes me apprehensive is any occasion that requires me to sit down *with* other people, usually to share a meal, for a set period of time.

Let's say I've been invited out for dinner. How long does the average restaurant booking last? About two hours? Maybe more? From the moment I'm asked to join the meal, I'll start thinking of it as something I have to get through. I'll consider ways out of it. Do I really need to go? Will it be frowned on if I decline? If I can't get out of it without being rude, I'll plan my coping strategies. Is there time for a run before I get there? Will alcohol be available? Will I be able to sit closer to the people I already know? Once I arrive, I'll assess the immediate threats. Is it too hot or noisy in the room? Are the lights too bright? It makes me uncomfortable when I can't quite hear what people are saying or when I'm in an airless room that makes my already overheating body get hotter and hotter. And for some reason, I feel exposed and squirmy when I sit beneath bright overhead lights. On their own or taken together, these things overstimulate me and dial my anxiety right up.

There was a time when I studiously avoided invitations to eat with my co-workers. I would pretend to have a meeting or an appointment to go to. When people in the office were getting ready to go have lunch or dinner together, I would disappear into the toilets and wait for 15 minutes until everyone had put their coats on and left through the front door. Then I'd creep out and leave through the back door.

Nowadays, I value every invitation that comes my way and make an effort to get involved. But I'm always fretting in advance about what the venue will be like.

The very worst setup for me? A small overcrowded restaurant with no air conditioning, where I'm crammed elbow-to-elbow with people who are meeting me for the first time under strong glaring lights — with no alcohol on the table. My least objectionable setup? A large restaurant with cool air or an al fresco space, sat with a handful of people I know in soft lighting – in the full knowledge there's enough alcohol within reach to keep my anxiety suppressed.

Alcohol played a forcible role early in my adult life but here's an idea of how it continues to shape my experiences. When I'm sat down for a meal with several people, I know exactly how much alcohol I'll need to settle my nerves. A single glass of wine is no good – exactly what you'll get if you order one bottle for the group – because it won't be enough to calm me down but it will be enough to make me feel hotter and encourage my skin to go red. I'll become conscious of the reddening and turn redder. (Alcohol stimulates vasodilation, making the capillaries in your face expand with blood. This happens to lots of people when they drink, but it's more or less a certainty if you blush easily.)

A single drink makes me more anxious because, once it's gone, I'll worry about getting the next one so I can put it into my system and get my mind to safety. Three, four or five drinks will soothe my anxiety and make me less likely to blush. So, having one drink and suddenly stopping doesn't work for me. I'd sooner avoid the single drink altogether. I'm much happier if I know the alcohol will be free-flowing. That way, I can refill my glass whenever I want. I'm fully aware it's an addictive attitude and a little too close to alcoholism for comfort.

I rely on booze because very often, when I sit at a table with other people, a sense of helplessness descends on me. I'm bound by social rules to sit and engage with my fellow diners and there are barely any means of escape. You can't stand up and leave a restaurant when simple interaction becomes too much for you. You can't retreat into an hour of stony silence when the conversation starts to overwhelm. To do these things is more than a little odd. It's outright anti-social. And because I want to be like everyone else enjoying good company and a sociable atmosphere, I bottle up my emotions and pretend they aren't swelling inside of me. It doesn't take long, maybe the first 20 or 30 minutes of the meal, for the pressure within to reach boiling point.

I engage for as long as I can. There comes a moment, though, especially in an animated, fast-talking group, when the stimulation on all sides overpowers me into silence. It's like hitting terminal velocity: I can't move any faster and just sitting at the table without running away now requires all of my effort. I have no surplus energy, there's nothing left to give, so I grow quiet and become an observer until someone notices I've dropped out of play and calls me out. *What do you think, Russell? Why are you so quiet?*

When my social anxiety spikes like this, I enter a kind of paralysis. It's like in the movies when a character is suddenly thrown into psychological turmoil. Let's say they've just witnessed a murder or learnt something life-changing. The camera will focus closely on them, edging out the rest of the world. All external noise will fade out, replaced by a low hum or a high ringing note. Time will slow down, the protagonist will start noticing small details in slow motion like someone's mouth shaping out silent words or light reflecting off a piece of jewellery. The overall effect is one of hyper-reality. The brain stalls and switches off its engines so it won't overheat, then floods with all the sensory input it would usually filter out as irrelevant. For that suspended moment, everything takes on a saturated quality. The minutiae of life throbs at maximum intensity. Then, when the shock wears off, the brain kicks into gear again and the character is suddenly 'back in the room' — usually to jump into action with a new-found sense of clarity.

When I'm stuck at the dinner table, especially without any alcohol, I don't slip into a hi-res coma or suddenly see the world in vivid Technicolor like I've eaten a bag of magic mushrooms. But time does begin to move very slowly so I'm acutely conscious of every passing second. I'll find myself looking down at my watch and focusing on the second hand, feeling it struggling to tick forwards, almost as though it wants to give up the fight and start travelling backwards. Has it really only been 60 seconds since I last looked at my watch? God, so much happens in a single minute. A conversation can start, a conversation can end, people can say so much and expect so much back and we've got 120 minutes or even more of this left to go. It's similar to being in pain, I suppose. When something hurts you physically, time takes on a new aspect. You notice time more keenly because it's not passive any more. It's measuring out your distress.

And that distress grows exponentially with the passage of time. My wife says my mouth starts twitching when I get nervous in a group. I purse my lips together with quick rhythmic jerks. This tiny facial tick, generally unobserved by everyone else, tells her I've started to struggle internally. As time grinds on and my anxiety builds, I eventually look for ways to get away from the table and blow off some steam. These days I don't smoke, so I can't use that excuse to disappear. The easiest option is a trip to the loo and so, during dinner, I tend to make two or three visits to the bathroom even when I don't need to go.

If there's no one else inside the gent's, I'll hover in front of the sinks and pretend to wash my hands while looking at my reflection in the mirror to check how red my face is. Otherwise, I'll lock myself inside a toilet stall (a recurring theme, you'll notice) and take deep breaths of the cool, damp air. I'll unbutton my shirt, close my eyes, press my face against the chilly porcelain tiles — anything to try to slow down my pulse and bring me back down to some semblance of reality. I'll stay away from the group until a good five or ten minutes tick past. Then I'll return slowly to the table, trying as hard as possible to keep my mind focused on other people and external things instead of my absurd internal reaction to them. Trying not to think about something is a contradiction in terms, of course, as you'll know if you've ever gone through a night of insomnia. (Making an effort not to think about something is still the act of thinking about it. The more you try to ignore being wide awake at 3am, the more awake you inevitably become.)

And so I stay permanently aware of my unease. The twitching lips lead to the surreptitious visits to the toilet and sooner or later, I start to close down and talk less. When people describe me, especially line managers I've had throughout my career, they use words like quiet, self-contained, considered, collected, calm. These are all polite ways of saying shy. Sometimes, people mistake this shyness for assurance. The less emotion they see, the more they assume you have it all under control. But they will never know how hard I'm trying, at all times, to process and suppress my emotions. I am not calm or collected or considered, I am wearing a precariously balanced mask and I live in constant fear of it falling off. It makes me feel like I lead a double life.

Some people would describe the workplace as a kind of double life. Your personal life and work life are two necessarily different things. I might be able to fall back on wine or beer at the dinner table but when I'm at work, there's nothing I can rely on beyond physical exercise and a good night's sleep to help me through a day full of nerves. And frequently these methods just aren't enough.

My career is dotted with crash-and-burn moments, when social anxiety took the reins out of my hands and ran its own reckless course. I remember a job interview at an advertising agency that was going really well until panic struck and I broke out in livid red blotches all over my face and neck. At the end, the interviewers told me bluntly that their clients would have no confidence in me face-to-face. So there was no second interview. I stood up in a workshop, once, to present a flipchart of ideas back to a roomful of participants. Halfway through my mind went utterly blank; the words were right there in front of me written down on paper, but I couldn't communicate them back to the group. I mumbled and sweated for a while, slowly drowning in adrenaline, until someone else mercifully took over. For a few months after that, I went under the office nickname 'Narcoleptic Norris'.

These moments of failure can feel like out-of-body experiences. You can't believe they're really happening, so part of you detaches from reality to watch from a safe distance. A catastrophe is happening to you, you are responding terribly to it, yet you are somehow separate from it all. When social anxiety hits me at its very hardest like this, I'm no longer aware of what I'm saying or doing. As far as I'm concerned, it's not me running the show any more. I've left the room and all I can do is watch passively as a man who looks like me goes up in a ball of self-inflicted flames. I watch it and I record it, because very soon it will be played back in my mind and pored over for many days to come.

If it sounds a little loopy described this way, it's even loopier when it happens to you. That's why I and anyone with Social Anxiety Disorder can end up spending a lifetime trying to avoid it at all costs. These crippling moments send us looking for crutches. Some people choose alcohol, some people choose nicotine. Others simply choose jobs and personal lives that let them keep a low profile. In my case, over the last decade or so, I've started taking beta blockers whenever I have a particularly stressful work event coming up.

Beta blockers are small pills that make a big difference. They're primarily designed to help patients recover from heart attacks, by regulating the body's blood pressure and stress hormones. But they have the secondary effect of blocking adrenaline in the sympathetic nervous system, which in turn makes anxious people feel calmer. I go to my doctor every once in a while to ask for a packet of Propranolol and the doctor happily prescribes them. On days when I have to present to clients, I keep one or two pills in my pocket and covertly swallow them about an hour before I need to step into action. It's hard to tell when they start working. Nothing really changes, I don't suddenly become confident and carefree, my personality doesn't shift from introvert to extrovert. But I do notice a very subtle dulling of the senses. Not of the mind, but of the senses: my hands tremble less, my skin feels cooler, I sweat less readily. At a molecular level, the adrenaline that fuels these nervous symptoms is being delicately regulated. My fight-or-flight response is being subdued. So I don't panic about panicking and for a brief moment (two pills last for about two hours) the cycle of social anxiety is broken. Finally, I can just get on with things without worrying about blushing, about twitching, about what other people are thinking about me.

Beta blockers helped me pass my driving test and give a speech at my wedding to more than 100 people. They've helped me make my way through interviews and presentations. When I use them, I feel liberated. But I choose the word 'use' here deliberately. There's always a downside to relying on medication like this. It might feel like you've finally found a cure but, by definition, a cure ends an illness. Beta blockers don't end social anxiety. They temporarily paper over the cracks. 'Don't treat the symptom, treat the cause' the famous saying goes. They're wise words but hard to live by.

It's possible to take too many beta blockers, to rely on them emotionally. I store them away like little nuggets of gold and ration them obsessively to make sure I always have enough on hand. *I've only got five doses left. Better use them wisely. There's that presentation at the end of January. Then there's the talk you're giving early in Feb. Keep them safe. Make every pill count.* When I have a few pills with me on the day I plan to use them, I keep putting my hand inside my pocket to feel their hard round edges and make sure they're still there.

It's addictive behaviour and I want to keep it in check. But I'm not always successful. If I ever find myself with a surplus of pills, the temptation to use them more often is hard to resist. At Christmas, for instance, I see a lot of family and friends and it's quite stressful. On Christmas Day, I will take some beta blockers 'just to take the edge off'. I will take some more on Boxing Day when I go out for dinner with my in-laws 'because it won't hurt'. And the truth is, it doesn't hurt. It helps me feel more relaxed and talkative and Christmas, on the whole, is more enjoyable as a result.

It's only afterwards that I sit back and ask myself why I need to swallow drugs to help me spend some time with my family. Slowly, it makes me feel bad. And the more I dwell on it, the worse I feel.

Rumination, of the deep and inwardly critical kind, completes the loop in the vicious cycle of social anxiety. It arrives soon after a perceived social failure, when you've escaped to solitude to sit and mull over what just happened to you. After all of the explosive over-stimulation, it feels like a heavy and distinct come-down. It, too, is something that all people with Social Anxiety Disorder want to avoid.

# 6. After

In the lead-up to a stressful social encounter, a small balloon, about the size of a grapefruit, swells deep in my stomach, straining against my body as it tries to escape up and outside into the open air. It's full of hormones and adrenaline and roiling nervous energy, all churning around and colliding, slowly generating heat and building up pressure. Why is the balloon there? Because of over-arousal. I am overstimulated by anticipation and worry and it has inflated itself in preparation for my fight or flight.

The balloon strains and strains, but it can't pop. It's only later, when I can retreat from the company of people to sit alone and recoup my senses, that it suddenly loses purpose and deflates. It leaves behind an empty, sinking feeling. Like it took a small part of me away with it.

A rush of adrenaline will always cause a crash. Just like a rush of serotonin, the brain's happy chemical, will always result in a comedown. An emotional peak creates an emotional trough. There's a name for it: dysphoria, the opposite of euphoria. It's a potent sense of dissatisfaction or unhappiness you can almost physically feel.

I feel it most keenly after a social encounter that went badly. I can feel the disappointment seeping from my stomach into my muscles and limbs. It makes me feel heavy and tired. And while my body decompresses, my mind starts to pick back over what has just happened – evaluating the damage sustained in over-magnified detail.

Here's a random case in point: I was once asked to come to an informal meeting to talk about proofreading. I have a qualification in proofreading (scouring through documents to mark up typos, grammatical slips, inconsistencies in style, etc) and the agency I worked for wanted to set up its own proofreading service. Could I attend the meeting and contribute at the end? Just to explain to the room exactly what proofreading was and why the agency needed it? That'll be fine, I thought. *It will only be the last five minutes of the meeting. Don't think about it in advance. Don't give it the chance to blow itself out of proportion. You know proofreading. You're on your own turf. Give it a quick top-level summary.* I could hear myself explaining it to other people in my mind. Short, measured, succinct. Just ignore the balloon, so it can't even inflate.

And that strategy worked in the run-up to the meeting. It was still working in the meeting itself as time wore on and my turn to speak drew near. *Just talk casually for five minutes. It's easy.* Then my boss said my name and handed the meeting over to me and every pair of eyes in the room turned to look in my direction. I was OK for the first 60 seconds or so. I defined proofreading and described my year-long training. Then I couldn't remember anything else I'd wanted to say. The balloon over-inflated and paralysed me. I fumbled my words and started ummm-ing and ahhh-ing. My sentences stopped having purpose and I started blurting out things about grammar, punctuation and syntax more or less at random. I started sweating, my mouth went dry, my voice tightened up.

Then I paused for breath and stopped talking, taking too long to formulate my next thought. Everyone sat perfectly still, looking to me to fill up a rapidly opening void.

Then a helpful soul said: 'I've heard it can be useful to read your work backwards. It makes it easier to spot your mistakes.' Someone else agreed, saying how hard it was to see errors in your own writing. Then someone said they wished they'd been taught grammar properly at school. And someone else said something about i before e except after c. One by one, people created their own conversation about proofreading while I sat there in silence. I still don't know if it was a natural ripple effect or if everyone was helping me out.

Then the five minutes were up and the meeting abruptly ended. Everyone filtered out of the room and I disappeared with them, out into the hallway, back up to my desk, where I sat down in my chair and stared at my computer screen. With something inside me quietly deflating.

If the event itself feels like a mental earthquake, then the aftermath – the recall, the scrutiny, the self-criticism – is a series of aftershocks. For the rest of that day, I felt downcast. I was certain I'd let myself down. I couldn't stop sifting through the wreckage of what, in my mind, had been a car crash: how certain people had looked at me, how others had looked at their watches, how some had avoided eye contact with me altogether, how one had frowned at me, how one had almost seemed to smile. I remember sitting on the train home that night, looking out at the masses of people waiting together on busy London platforms, wondering how impossible it was to know what's going on in other people's minds. And crucially, what other people were thinking about you and the way you behaved. It stuck with me for the rest of that week, the next few months and throughout the rest of the year. Then the year after that. Even when I write about it now, several years later, it makes me cringe.

All of this fallout from five minutes that took place so long ago. Why does the memory persist so strongly, staying with me? Why do any of these stressful episodes? In this particular case (one of thousands I've obsessed over thus far in my life) it's because it made me step back to look at my personality and ask myself questions like these:

Does my boss think there's something wrong with me? She asked me to speak for a few minutes and I imploded in front of everyone, she must think I have some real social issues that make me unfit for my job. Will she start behaving differently around me now, or even suggest that I go get some help with public speaking? What was everyone thinking when the spotlight went on me and I couldn't talk confidently for five minutes? Were they thinking I'm not very good at what I do? Were they wondering if I always crumble like this? Were they thinking I'm a little bit strange? Were they embarrassed for me? Were they thinking: 'Wow, five minutes and he lost the plot, at least I'm not as bad as this guy.' Were they secretly laughing at me? When everyone walked out of the room at the very end, did they roll their eyes and smile and whisper to each other: 'Jesus, what was that? I could barely watch!' Did this opinion of me then attach itself permanently to their minds, so whenever they pass me in the hallway now or see me in the canteen or sit with me in a meeting, they see me as the guy who's always on edge and socially awkward to be around? Does it make them not want to talk to me, not want to be in my presence – does it ultimately make them dislike me? What do they really think about me?

The truth is, we can never fully know ourselves without knowing how others see us. When we're judged or evaluated by another person, it becomes part of our own opinion of ourselves. People are so intrinsic to our identity, we cannot complete the puzzle of who we are without them.

Living in a world where other human beings are thinking about you – and never being able to know what those external thoughts are – is a perpetual torment. It's the myth of Sisyphus; a king doomed for eternity to roll a boulder up a hill only to see it roll back down again. Or the story of Tantalus; a mortal banished to the underworld, where food and water would always remain just beyond his grasp. It's a state of futility, a recurring problem that is never resolved.

After an overwhelming social event, socially anxious people sit alone and try to make sense of themselves through other people's eyes.

But we simply can't do it. Nobody can. It's impossible to truly assess yourself from the outside. And that's why most people, quite rationally, are less disposed to see the rest of the world as an audience that's watching them. But social anxiety turns all eyes, everywhere, in your direction. It creates an artificial audience that you know can't be real, yet you nonetheless carry around with you wherever you go.

When you feel so keenly that all other people are primed to watch you, to examine you, to judge you, it can feel very much like you're dragging a ball and chain around with every step. Just like those ancient Greek myths, the experience has all the qualities of a very personal punishment.

So it's no wonder that every poor social encounter makes someone with SAD question their whole personality and every aspect of their lives. Even though they know that people probably aren't assessing them half as much as they feel they are. There's a fine line between social phobia and paranoia, but it's an important line to acknowledge. A phobia is irrational but it doesn't try to place any blame: I might fear other people but I don't hold them responsible for my distress. Paranoia is irrational too but it tells a different story. If I were clinically paranoid, I'd be convinced that everyone is watching me because they're all trying to distress me on purpose. Paranoia means you know that everyone is conspiring against you. Social phobia means you know that you're conspiring against yourself.

Social anxiety flows through a cycle, before, during and after any agitating human contact. It starts with stage fright, peaks with panic and concludes with dysphoria. And because it was unpleasant and you don't want to go through it again, your fear increases every time the cycle reboots.

And so on.

And so on.

And so on.

But remember: with every curse comes a blessing. If Social Anxiety Disorder creates three distinct shades of unhappiness, we should also recognise that the opposite feeling – happiness – is perceived in three distinct ways too. Before happiness comes the anticipation of it, then the experience of it and finally the recall. Because it was pleasant and you want to go through it again, you look forward to it more and more. Perhaps this self-fulfilling force is more natural than we think. Take it away from sadness and you might have to take it away from happiness, too.

# 7: Origin

So much of social anxiety boils down to two intrinsic factors: genetics and environment. While I don't believe we can adequately explain away our adulthood by evaluating our childhood, our earliest years can significantly influence who we later become.

The argument at play here is the infamous question of nature versus nurture. Broadly speaking, it suggests that either one or the other shapes you as a person. If you side with nature, you believe that people behave the way they do because it was written in their biological make-up from birth. If you side with nurture, you believe that life begins as a blank slate for everyone and our upbringing and education dictates our behaviour.

There's a third angle that suggests it's not nature or nurture working independently, but both factors working together in a

50/50 mix. And that's the idea that makes most sense to me, if I peer into my past. Nature built the framework and nurture fleshed it out.

So let's start with the framework, the genetic blueprint that nature selects for you (and only you) to make you who you are. That means starting with a brief sketch of my parents.

My dad grew up in Wimbledon, South London, one of three children who came of age in the 1960s. He showed early athletic ability at school, particularly in swimming. As he entered his teens he was competing in swimming galas for his county, Surrey, and by his mid-teens he'd broken the UK record for the 110-yards Butterfly. His record of 57.2 seconds lasted for five years, long enough to attract the interest of an American college. Oklahoma State University offered him a full educational scholarship and he was entered into the 1968 Mexico Olympics (though he couldn't compete because of food poisoning). It was while he was swimming and studying in Oklahoma that he met my mother.

My mother was born in a small Oklahoman town surrounded by spinach farms and pastureland. She was one of eight children in a family with some Native American heritage that showed an inclination towards music. Her older brother would later become a talented pianist and the leader of B Bumble & The Stingers, an instrumental rock band with a string of hits in the 1960s. My mum would get in front of a microphone and sing three-part harmonies with her sisters at parties and began learning the piano from a young age.

My dad has always been good with numbers and he majored in Computer Mathematics. My mum was always interested in literature and the arts, so she majored in the Humanities. Soon after graduation, they got married and started a family. My sister came first and then, a year later, my mum gave birth to me.

I mention all of these details – the British side vs the American side, the swimming vs the music, the maths vs the arts – because they highlight how different my parents are. My mum loves Mozart and Chopin and plays piano every Sunday at her church. My dad likes Jimi Hendrix and Fleetwood Mac and has no interest in church. My mum likes to sit quietly and read a good book, while my dad prefers to sit and watch a loud action movie. My mum is not competitive. My dad likes to win. My mum is an introvert. My dad is an extrovert. They naturally complement each other.

But where do these differences begin? What made my dad my dad and my mum my mum? Learning an instrument, following a religion, preferring to read stories on the page instead of watching stories on the screen: you can argue these are behaviours and tastes they each acquired through exposure (or the lack of it). These are the products of nurture and environment and we aren't necessarily born with them. But we are born with a Left Brain and a Right Brain and one side always seems to dominate over the other.

The Right Brain is considered the more creative and artistic half. It's adept at reading or expressing emotions, understanding music, appreciating colours, harnessing the imagination and showing intuition. It helps us act on stage, play a violin, paint a picture, tell a story. The Left Brain is more analytical and critical. It's proficient at language, numbers, logic and reasoning. It helps us to learn a new language, calculate equations or make sense of data. We all use both sides of our brain every day but we all show a natural preference for the Left or the Right. My dad, I would say, is Left-Brained. And my mum is Right-Brained. I consider myself Right-Brained, too. As we grow, this predominance goes on to inform our choices in ways we're unaware of, giving nature and biology a truly pivotal role in our lives.

The biological differences between my mum and dad are equally definitive. Before he went grey my father had fair hair and he's always had typically pale, typically English skin. As a boy, his face would freckle up in the summertime and burn fast. I presume it's where my sensitive skin comes from. I seem to have picked up most of my father's physical attributes and missed out on a lot of the characteristics from my mother's gene pool. By contrast, she used to have jet-black hair and would tan quickly as a young woman. When I look at photos of her as a teenager, baked deep brown by the fierce Midwestern sun, she looks Spanish or almost Mexican and not at all a woman whose family could trace its roots back to Scottish immigrants in the 19th century.

I always see myself as British through and through. Not just biologically but psychologically, too. I look British, courtesy of nature. And I think in a thoroughly British way, courtesy of nurture. So it always feels strange to think that I spent my earliest years as an American.

The first house my parents lived in as a married couple was a bungalow in the suburbs of Tulsa, Oklahoma. I came along in 1980. My dad tells me I cried a lot as a baby. My mum tells me I was prone to illness. Both seem typical for a small child. But they insist I was more sensitive, to more or less everything, than my sister. I caught the Coxsackie virus as a baby and it filled up my mouth and throat with blisters. I always seemed to have colic. When I came down with the chicken pox, every inch of my skin went into revolt: pustules popped up all over my body, from inside my ears to in between my toes. Sudden movements or sounds would startle me. I only wanted to be held by my mother and would cry when handed to anyone else.

My mum has a clear recollection of me, about eight months old, crawling around the living room to explore the bookshelves, the chair legs, the radiators, anything within reach. She had a number of potted plants in the house, including one with long trailing stems that hung down as low as the carpet. I would regularly make a beeline for this plant and try to yank off a few leaves. On this occasion, my mum saw me from across the room and cut me off at the pass. She called out my name with a rising intonation at the end. She remembers it because the change in tone was subtle, the kind of thing my sister would ignore. But as soon as I heard my name with that new tone, I froze in my tracks, turned round to look at my mum as though my universe had imploded — and launched into a long crying fit.

My dad remembers something from a little later, when I was almost two years old. The street we lived on was full of identical houses, all of them mock-fieldstone bungalows that sat long and low in a carefully landscaped estate. Every house had one big lawn that surrounded it on all sides. There was no front garden or back garden or any fences to mark where one property ended and another began. There were just wide open stretches of stiff, sun-baked grass — one continuous playground for all the local children. The more fun stuff you had in your backyard (trampolines, climbing frames, slides) the more kids stopped by to play with you. We were still new to the area and my dad was keen for my sister and I to make more friends our age. So he bought a complicated swing set and spent a long weekend screwing it all together. Sure enough, when some neighbouring kids noticed this new novelty, they came over to our lawn in their dozens, but only my sister would play with them. I would back away from the group and watch them all playing from the safe distance of our back porch. My sister and the local children got on like a house on fire and she soon ran off with them to other lawns and toys.

And then comes the image that stuck in my dad's mind. The next time he looked out of the window to check on us, everyone was gone except for me. I'd ventured back out to the swing set and was sitting on one side of a see-saw designed for two children, trying to swing back and forth on my own. He says he felt conflicted because on one hand he was sad to see me missing out on all the fun. But on the other hand, I seemed much happier sitting out there alone: 'Even then, you liked your solitude.'

Ultimately, it would make no difference if we made new friends in Tulsa. In 1982, my dad got a job offer that brought him back to England. The move was always a temporary plan but the more time we spent with old friends, the more permanent it became.

# 8. Dogma

When we arrived back in the UK my parents settled in south London, in an old semi-detached house in Morden. Opposite the house was a large concrete car park that was always empty on weekends. I remember spending long hours in this car park with my sister, learning how to ride our bicycles. It was surrounded on all sides by a tall chain-link fence. And that pleased me, because there were always lots of dogs in the area and the fence kept them out. Wherever we went, there were dogs: being walked on the street, running loose in the park, tied up to lampposts or rails outside shops. Or perhaps that's just the way it seemed.

Just around the corner from our house was a video rental store. It's funny to think of it now but not so very long ago, if you wanted to watch a decent movie you had to browse through thousands of video cassettes lined up in rows on shelves. We went to this place often, usually as a family outing on Friday nights, to pick up some new movies for the weekend.

One visit to this shop stands out vividly. I had wandered away from my parents and my sister and was scanning the endless spines of VHS boxes, looking for He-Man, Transformers and Danger Mouse. I must have been close to the shop door because I heard a bell tinkle as someone pushed it open and came inside. I saw a man pull a dog into the store and casually unclip its leash. I froze on the spot, watching this giant, muscular animal loudly licking its lips.

What kind of dog was it? Maybe a labrador or a retriever. I have no idea but it seemed colossal at my eye level. Colossal, too, was the threat it posed. The dog was circling round excitedly, scratching its feet against the carpet and flicking its tail against video boxes. It looked like it might do anything at any moment. I suddenly became very aware that my mum and dad had drifted out of sight and I wanted them here right now, more than anything, to form a barrier between me and the dog just a few feet away.

Of course, at that moment, the dog's ears pricked up and it whirled around to look at me. My dad would later tell me that dogs can smell fear, so the best thing to do is never be afraid of them.

The only thing to do was run away. I flew blindly down aisles of videos, not stopping to consider left or right but just sprinting as fast as I could to get away from the dog, who was bounding behind me. The shop floor started to feel like a maze, one corridor leading to the next and every time I turned a corner I felt more and more lost. Looking back on this now makes me laugh – a little boy fleeing from a curious dog, but at the time it had all the cinematic gravity of something from *Alien*. I was being stalked down unfamiliar passageways by a monster who would stop at nothing to rip me to pieces. In the video shop, no one can hear you scream. I was so frightened that I couldn't even cry out. I'd lost my breath and all I could feel was my heart thumping deep down in my throat. And then, right on cue, I ran straight down an aisle that came to a dead end.

I pressed my back flat against the wall and watched the dog bound into view at the far end. Again, the level of terror flooding my world made everything seem like a movie. When I saw *Ghostbusters* for the first time, the scene where Slimer charges at Venkman down a hotel hallway echoes this memory. The same goes for *Jurassic Park*, when the Raptors chase kids through rows of industrial kitchen units. I stood there in horror as the dog sprang into action and ran full-pelt towards me, racing closer and closer until it jumped up on its hind legs and threw its paws on my shoulders and my face disappeared into a slobbering maw of teeth.

I think my voice returned, at that point, and I screeched out for help. All of a sudden my dad was leading me away by the hand, the dog was trotting off and I was back alongside my mum and my sister who were totally oblivious to the nightmare I'd lived through.

For a long time after this, I hated dogs. I would cross the street to avoid them. I wouldn't go into the park if they were running around. And whenever we went to a dog-owners house, my parents would either politely ask our hosts to shut the dogs away in another room or I would spend the entire visit sitting like a stone statue next to my mum or dad, not daring to move a muscle in case I made the dogs aware of my existence.

I believe this was my first ever act of avoidance.

I'd later outgrow this fear. But for some people, well into adulthood, fear of dogs is persistent. It's called *cynophobia* and sits in a special subcategory of 'animal phobias'. Aversion to a particular kind of animal is common. Most people will admit to disliking one creature or another. Usually snakes, spiders, slugs, worms or anything creepy-crawly. People with *arachnophobia* get worried before they even see a spider. They actively avoid anywhere that might conceal one, living in a permanent state of high alert. The anxiety of when, where and how they might encounter their most dreaded fear builds and builds and builds. So that when they finally do, the experience hits them a hundredfold. *You can never go through that ordeal again* declares their phobia, when the moment of pure horror has mercifully passed. And their private campaign to keep away from spiders at all costs doubles its energy.

Does that sound familiar? I hope you can see the parallels.

In 1971, the psychologist Stanley Rachman suggested that, to be indelibly acquired, a fear has to meet three conditions. The first is direct personal experience: you once had a bad encounter with a dog, possibly because it bit you. The second is observational experience: you once saw someone else attacked or upset by a dog. The third is instructional experience: you were once warned to avoid dogs because they might hurt you (and this in turn probably came from someone who'd been through the same three stages of experience).

A phobia creates an inner world that revolves around the object of your fear and everything in it feels personalised. But viewed with a little perspective, it starts to look like our capacity for phobia is pre-prepared. All we need to do is meet the right criteria, tick the right neural boxes, and a phobia springs up from our subconscious ready-made. So why wasn't it dogs for me, instead of people? Why wasn't it spiders or aeroplanes or germs or buttons? If three conditions help a phobia take root, can I trace three specific memories that fit into this theory?

Firstly, we have direct personal experience. While living in Morden, I joined a local nursery. My recollections are hazy but the harder I try to look back, the more I start to see a few isolated incidents. The school had a small bathroom, built for small people. Mini urinals on the wall and mini toilets in mini cubicles. I was mini too, of course, but I somehow knew these things had been made especially for us. And for that reason, the bathroom felt like a safe place. It was quiet in there. And going to the toilet alone gave you a sense of achievement. I remember sitting on a toilet, doing my thing, enjoying the closed-off feeling of a locked toilet stall. Then I heard the bathroom door bang open and lots of shoes clapping against the hard tiles on the floor. I heard some kids yanking open the cubicle doors on either side of me and jumping up onto toilet seats. Before I knew it, four or five laughing faces appeared over the top of my stall. Hands were pointing at me and voices were calling me smelly, dirty, yucky, disgusting.

I remember a feeling of absolute exposure. There I was, scrambling to pull my pants up, under fire from all sides. It was invasive. And cosmically unfair. Why was this suddenly happening to me? How could other people be allowed to do this? They were older kids, I think, and they weren't supposed to be in the smaller toilets. Before long they'd jumped down and run away out into the corridor, leaving the bathroom door swinging on its hinges. I stayed on the toilet for a little while, with my pants and trousers back on, worried they'd come back in at any minute. And I think for the first time ever I felt a genuine sense of shame.

Is that enough to spark a phobia of people? I'm sure everyone has a few memories like that. The next stage is observational experience. At this age, I must have been three or four, did I ever witness something socially traumatic happening to somebody else? Maybe. Every year at my nursery, we had an Easter bonnet competition. Children would create their own Easter hats at home with their parents, then bring them in for a parade-style ceremony in the nursery gym. Some kids turned up with elaborate works of art on their heads. Lots of curly paper ribbons in springtime colours, carefully strewn through tufts of fake grass. Lots of fake baby chicks and papier mache eggs delicately glued together. In retrospect, the whole event was one big display of one-upmanship for the parents. And some parents either didn't know how to or simply couldn't be bothered to play the game.

Every kid had to do a lap of the gym wearing their Easter bonnet, while the nursery staff sat in a row like a panel of judges. Everyone was desperate to claim the prize for best bonnet. Interestingly enough, I have no recollection of my own bonnet or my journey round the gym in front of all those judgemental eyes. But I do remember one kid who didn't have an Easter hat. Instead, he had an empty cereal box on top of his head, cut into the shape of a crown. It was a rubbish-looking hat and lots of children started to giggle as he stepped to the front of the parade queue. He obviously didn't want to go through with it and started crying almost immediately. He made his way around the gymnasium in floods of humiliated tears, while scores of parents, children and teachers watched. I took a clear message away from that, just as I'm sure the rest of the nursery did: never be the kid without the Easter bonnet. Which essentially means never be the odd one out. Because you'll draw unwanted attention. And it will make you feel sad.

What about the third and final stage, instructional experience? I watched a lot of cartoons, growing up. Disney's *Robin Hood* came out well before my time in 1973 but by 1984, when I was getting closer and closer to primary school, it was on TV a lot. Or else it was playing in our VCR a lot. I remember one character in the film called Toby Turtle, who spoke slowly and methodically and approached everything in the world with gentle caution. The rest of his young friends were happy-go-lucky rabbits, who considered him a bit of a wet blanket. Toby would watch his pals get into daring scrapes from the safety of the sidelines. He shied away from confrontation, retreating into his shell whenever he felt scared or threatened. There's one scene where the rabbits gang up on him because they're worried he'll tell their parents they've been up to no good. They consider him weak-willed and a natural liability. So they make him swear an oath as they all stand around him in a ring: 'If I tattle-tale, I'll die until I'm dead.'

It was all done in good humour and Disney were obviously playing with stereotypes: bold vs timid, loud vs quiet, brave vs cowardly and so on. But I remember feeling instinctively sorry for Toby. Everything about him was tinged with sadness. His face, his voice, his personality. Whenever he was on-screen I wanted to cry on his behalf. Because his sadness came from the creatures all around him. They were the ones who made him feel insecure and he was retreating from them when he shrank back inside his shell. There were loads of cartoon characters on TV who fell into this camp. Piglet in Winnie-the-Pooh was always nervous and worried. Porky Pig in Looney Tunes was vulnerable because of his stutter. Charlie Brown in Peanuts was dominated by his fear of rejection. These were the emotional caricatures I was drawn to. And the unspoken advice they seemed to send out was: beware the judgement of others.

But there were equal if not greater numbers of self-assured, confident, assertive characters out there too. Characters who usually took on the role of the hero. Why didn't they make more of an impression? Perhaps something inside me was already primed for observation and preservation, instead of action and risk. Just like a pre-formed phobia, lying in wait for the right mental stimulus to come along and get trapped under its lens. Once a fear is imprisoned and magnified there, it becomes a psychological truth that imprisons you with it.

It all makes me think of the torture chamber in Orwell's *1984*. Do you remember how that dystopian novel comes to an end? Winston Smith, a rebel in a totalitarian state, is sent to Room 101, which contains everyone's worst fear. Everyone knows what's inside that room because everyone has a singular dread. 'For everyone there is something unendurable — something that cannot be contemplated.' In Winston's case, rats are the very worst thing in the world. And when he's strapped into a chair, with a cage full of starving rodents about to be lowered onto and locked around his head, he finally breaks — physically, mentally, spiritually — and commits the ultimate act of avoidance. He begs his torturers to inflict the same punishment on someone else, in return for his total obedience.

Perhaps by choosing rats, Orwell was demonstrating the uncontrollable nature of a fear that runs all over you.

Just about everything is uncontrollable when you're an infant. And what makes a phobia so distressing as an adult is the way that uncontrollable world can suddenly revisit you. Every time I feel socially anxious, I feel the helplessness of a child. It's like reaching back across three decades to the unadulterated source of my fear. I want to know what that source was, and is. So let's keep looking for it.

# 9. Sink or swim

As I made my way through primary school, I was encouraged to take up swimming. This was inevitable, I suppose, given my dad's background. But it started at first with simple lessons for everyone at school. My whole class would jump into the local swimming baths and thrash, float or doggy-paddle their way to a new swimming badge. The 10m badge became the 15m badge became the 20m badge. And before long, I was comfortably mucking about in the water with the rest of my age group.

I was soon taking lessons outside of school, one night a week, with a personal coach. She taught me the basics of each stroke — front crawl, breaststroke, butterfly and backstroke — and watched for an inclination towards one or the other. It turned out I was better at backstroke, so we focused on that.

I was always nervous before these swimming lessons. Nervous because the coach wanted to see improvement week on week and I wanted to please her, nervous because I knew my dad was watching and I wanted to make him proud, nervous because the swimming baths had a public viewing gallery with lots of people looking down on the swimmers below. The building was old and imposing. In the foyer there were green marble floors that echoed when you walked across them and made you feel small. Above the pool, there was a high domed roof that mixed together a constant cocktail of sound: parents chatting to each other, trainers blowing their whistles, kids shouting to each other, water splishing and splashing as swimmers tried to perfect their dives and turns. It all merged together into one deep, cavernous hum. Like the restless murmur of an expectant crowd.

These nerves hadn't become 'bad' nerves just yet. They were the kind of nerves that some people might even call good. I was excited by the bright lights and the noise and the physical activity, by the encouragement and attention I was getting from my teacher and my dad. I now know that this was more than a state of excitement. It was a state of over-arousal. Although I had no idea of this distinction. It even felt beneficial at first, being totally alert and ready for anything. You often hear athletes praising the power of pre-race nerves, calling it a special buzz that enhances your performance. Those are the 'good' nerves that prove you care deeply about your sport.

But over-aroused quickly becomes overwhelmed. And those good nerves turned bad, for me, as soon as I started to compete. After a year or so, my teacher entered me into a series of galas. I swam as part of a team in medleys at first, then competed on my own in the backstroke. I would constantly fret about these races, counting down the days until the scheduled date arrived. And on the morning of the competition I would feel sick, almost wishing I was sick with the measles or the chickenpox so I could stay in bed all day and avoid the whole thing.

But I always went. Once we arrived at the baths, my dad would disappear upstairs into the packed viewing gallery and I would file into the damp changing rooms with scores of chattering kids. And when I walked out pool-side into the hot air that buzzed with noise and stung my nostrils with chlorine, the sense of doom was absolute.

Most races began with a loud bang from the starter's pistol. And I started to fear that moment almost as much as the race itself. I hated how jittery it made me. When I was sitting on the sidelines watching the other races begin, at least I could secretly put my fingers in my ears. But there was no chance of doing that up on the blocks. And so I worried about it more and more as my swim drew closer. And then when my turn came, I hated waiting for that gun to go off, feeling wound-up and twitchy and praying I wouldn't jump too early and give a false start. I'd be entirely focused on the gun instead of the swimming. When's it gonna go? Not yet, not yet, not yet. And when it finally went off with an almighty crack, I would flinch or shudder and waste a precious half-second before snapping into action.

There was one time when I'd been entered into the 100m backstroke. My family was up in the gallery, along with some of my teachers from school. I was swimming for Surrey County at that point and the pressure had gone up. You always start the backstroke in the water and I remember being curled up into a ball, my hands gripping the edge of the floor tiles and my feet pressed flat against the wall of the pool. The starter called 'set' and I curled up even tighter, ready to let loose like a spring. Then came the interminable wait for the explosion from the pistol, long drawn-out seconds with my teeth gritted hard and my eyes screwed shut.

When the gun echoed all around the swimming hall, I flew away from the wall in one of my best starts ever. I swang my arms and pumped my legs, sending clear blue water flying up in all directions. The sound of the crowd came to me in snatches as my head dipped in and out of the water. Through my foggy goggles, I saw one of my teachers leaning over the railings up in the gallery, waving her fists and cheering me on. I looked left and right: I was in first place and it felt like I had a big lead. So I swam with every muscle, pulling as hard as I could, until I saw a familiar string of coloured flags passing by overhead.

These flags tell swimmers on their backs how far they are from the finish. You're supposed to know, from your practice swims, how many strokes are left from the flags to the end of the pool. But for me, this was never an exact science. The number of strokes was always changing, especially on race days. Many times, I had trusted a set number — and ungracefully ended my race by smashing my arm or the back of my head into the ceramic edge of the pool. I was scared of doing it again and so, as I neared the end of the lane, I slowed down and turned my neck to one side, so I could see the pool edge coming towards me. Then I glided to a finish and won the race.

Or at least, that's what I thought until someone told me to step away from the winner's podium. A marshal explained to me that I'd turned over during my finish, which was illegal. I'd been disqualified and the kid in second place got the golden trophy.

I was devastated and spent the rest of the competition sitting on a bench, unable to look up at the seats in the gallery to meet my dad's eye. I think that was when, for the first time, he realised how much these competitions were rattling me. Because later that night, back at home before bedtime, he came into my room and asked me if I genuinely enjoyed swimming and if I wanted to keep on doing it. Through tears, I told him it wasn't fun and it made me feel sick. So the training and the galas stopped. And I felt a full-body sense of relief.

A bit later, when I was seven or eight years old, I started taking piano lessons. My mother knew a retired lady at church who taught local children after school. Her name was Mrs Norman and from her very first visit I found her terrifying. Partly, I think, it was her appearance. At some point she'd suffered a stroke and one side of her face had completely frozen. Her mouth on the affected side drooped downwards and she spoke through it sideways, in a clipped and straining voice that I sometimes struggled to understand. Her eye on that side was expressionless. It would stare at you coldly and critically, never blinking. She had to dab it dry every few minutes with a handkerchief. But how she looked isn't what scared me the most. That fear was reserved for how she taught.

Mrs Norman was frighteningly old-school. Her accent came from a different time and place. Pure BBC English, delivered with military purpose. She had no time for small talk. When she arrived at our house, she would almost brush my mum aside with her walking stick as she strode down the hallway and into the dining room. That's where we kept our piano: a beautiful, black, upright Bechstein. She would draw up a chair at the end of the keyboard, pull out some song sheets from her oversized handbag and wait impatiently for either me or my sister to enter the room, shut the door behind us and take our place on the piano stool.

My sister usually had her lesson first. For 30 minutes I'd sit and wait in the living room, listening to halting melodies and muffled reprimands from Mrs Norman on the other side of the wall. And all that waiting was interminable. I would watch the clock ticking steadily forward, switch on the TV to try and distract myself, go upstairs and waste a few minutes in the bathroom. In there I ran my hands under the cold taps, because they were hot and sweaty and slippery fingers always made my piano-playing worse. I knew when the lesson was drawing to a close because it would go quiet in the dining room. Mrs Norman was writing down some homework for the next week in a large, unsteady hand. And my sister was probably swinging her legs under her stool, glad to be finished. She didn't like the lessons any more than I did, but somehow they didn't affect her so much.

I'd be a quivering wreck by this point. My mum would stick her head into the living room and nod, which was my signal to go out into the hallway and wait. My sister would exit the dining room and give me a knowing grimace. And I would watch the door swing back shut, knowing that Mrs Norman was now sitting there with her steely eye, waiting for me to get my act together and come into the room. I can picture this moment clearly, delaying outside the door, wishing the ground would open up and swallow me or that I could somehow pause time forever and never have to go through with the lesson. I would blow air onto my clammy palms to try and dry them off. And the air all around me would grow thick and heavy with silence. (In all likelihood, this is where my fear of entering rooms began.) Every week it seemed to get harder but there was no way around it. The moment always came when I had to grip the doorknob and face up to 30 minutes of scrutiny from my petrifying piano teacher.

And maybe that's why I always found it so hard, because the very nature of a lesson means you have to perform while being watched. I've always performed below my ability when people watch me do something. Even now, as an adult, when I have to do something while being observed, I lose my focus. And that's how these piano lessons always played out for me. Half an hour of repeatedly losing my focus.

Mrs Norman was tough. She believed in drills, regimented practice, playing a passage over and over and over until it was drummed into you and you could play it off by heart. I struggled to read sheet music. She would explain to me, again and again, the difference between whole notes, crotchets and quavers. And when to rest between notes or hold them. And when a note is sharp, flat or natural. But translating these symbols from the page to my fingertips was very difficult for me. Learning to read music is like learning to read a new language. My brain was very slow to compute. Not least because it was more concerned with performance anxiety.

But Mrs Norman didn't believe in performance anxiety. She believed in progress, week by week. And steadily passing your grade exams. When I messed up midway through a simple piece of music, staring down at the keyboard for some clue how to continue, she would order me to start again. And when I faltered again, even earlier in the piece, she'd angrily take the sheet music away from me and command me through basic scales and exercises for the rest of the lesson. And I would leave that lesson feeling like a failure.

Looking back on this, I understand her logic. When you fail a task, you repeat that task until you complete it successfully. That's how you improve, so that's exactly what we did. But for months on end I didn't improve. I reached a certain level and failed to move forwards, much to her frustration and disappointment. I don't think it ever crossed her mind that my failure could be caused by anything other than inability. (Very often, when I was practising piano alone, I made my way through the same music – and more complicated music – with no mistakes at all.)

In the end, Mrs Norman decided I had learning difficulties. It was a glib misjudgement to aim at a kid. She told my mother the piano wasn't for me and perhaps I needed some special attention at school. This time, it was my mum's turn to come to my bedroom that night and ask me if I really enjoyed playing the piano. And if I wanted to carry on. Again, through tears, I told her I hated it and I hated Mrs Norman even more. So the lessons stopped and I never had another one again.

But the truth is, I didn't hate the piano. And I didn't hate swimming. Recreationally, with no strings attached, I enjoyed them both. What I hated was being put under social pressure. I wish I'd known how to identify the true cause of my nerves, growing up. Because if I had, I might have found a sport I loved to play. And I may have mastered a musical instrument. Instead, I decided that both of these things made me feel bad and I was better off avoiding them.

The other week, I went back to my parents' house and sat down at the same black Bechstein. Without thinking about it, I put my hands on the keys, shut my eyes and played a tricky little song called the Gypsy Tango. It was the one song that Mrs Norman made me practise the most, because I always screwed it up. This time, though, I played it perfectly.

Somewhere in a dusty recess of my younger brain, that music made a home for itself and stayed there. Now it was transferring itself effortlessly to my fingertips, in a way it never did when I was being forced to play it. So, as it turns out, I can play the piano. But just that one song. And I play it best alone.

# 10. Anglo-American

Just about every year in the lead-up to my teens, we went back to America to spend long summer holidays with my mum's side of the family. School would finish and we'd catch a jumbo jet to Dallas, Texas – then get on a tiny rattling propeller plane to Fort Smith, Arkansas. Air travel excited me but I wasn't a fan of take-offs and landings. Those tense moments on the runway sent a familiar prickle of nerves creeping through my body. I'd get hot and sweaty and turn my air-con up to the max. The stewardesses on American Airlines made me feel uncomfortable, too. They always wanted to talk about where I was going and who I'd see there. They wore lots of makeup and called me little man or sweetheart and told me my accent was cute. I was awkward around them and relieved when their trolley finally moved on down the aisle, so the stilted conversations would stop.

From Fort Smith it was an hour's drive across the state border into Oklahoma, where my grandparents lived on the edge of a tiny town called Spiro. A tiny town, perhaps, but my grandparents' house was enormous. The front porch was high and monolithic, supported by big white colonial-style pillars. Out back was a huge swimming pool with a diving board and a built-in water slide. To the side of the house was a basketball court and a garage where my grandad parked his pick-up trucks and a quad bike. All around, for miles and miles right up to the shimmering horizon, there was nothing but sun-soaked pastureland dotted with groups of grazing cattle.

It was far from cramped, rainy London. And I always felt the difference keenly. Most keenly when we were playing with my American cousins. They were usually brown all over from hours spent outside in the Midwestern sunshine. The Oklahoman summers are brutal. The sun beats down hard for weeks on end, hitting 38°C and higher. When we all went out swimming in the glimmering pool, my cousins would splash around in their bathing suits and top up their tans. My mum always slathered me in factor 50 suncream and made me wear a hat and t-shirt, even in the water. Despite the protection, by the end of the day parts of me would still be sunburnt. And I'd spend the evening lying prone on the sofa, while my mum dabbed cold calamine lotion over my calves or across the back of my neck.

The grass in Oklahoma isn't like English grass. It's sharp and scratchy and it hurt my feet when I ran across it. My cousins had hard, calloused feet and it didn't bother them in the slightest. They had scars on their bodies too, from falling off horses or carelessly chopping wood. But beyond a grazed elbow or knee I'd never been injured in any way. The mosquitoes didn't go after them at night-time in their bedrooms. But I would wake up each morning with big, swollen mozzie bites in really awkward places. On my knuckles, in my ears, all around my ankles and feet. My cousins were gung-ho and outspoken in a way I'd never experienced at home. I was painfully aware of the gap between their way of life and mine. And that gap got even bigger when I stepped outside our family circle.

There are lots of stereotypes about Americans. Americans talk too much; Americans talk too loud; Americans are aggressively extrovert. At heart, I think most Americans are just welcoming and generous. But to outsiders it can sometimes feel like a brand of optimism that's stuck in overdrive. There were certainly times when I struggled with it during my summers there.

Because everyone wanted to talk to me. And I mean everyone. Every storekeeper at every checkout, every waiter in every restaurant. Car park attendants, cleaners in bathrooms, total strangers who saw I was dressed differently or overheard my accent and came over to start asking questions. Where I was from. Why I was here. How I liked things over here in the U-S-of-A. And a 20-minute conversation would begin, making it impossible to go anywhere or do anything without becoming the centre of attention. Which was the one thing I didn't want to be.

I found it unsettling in clothes stores, when a sales assistant would come over and ask for my name, then address me personally for the rest of the time I spent in the shop. They'd bring me different items to try on without being asked and call out to me through the changing room door: 'Hey Russell, how ya gettin' on in there?' I would hide on the other side and take longer than I needed to get dressed, wishing the voice on the outside would just leave me alone so I could do my own shopping in peace. I think I knew, by this age, that social interaction — and particularly small talk — pushed me into a state of retreat. And being confronted by that fear all day long was draining.

So naturally I started to avoid it. I would make my mum come into shops with me and do all the talking. Or I'd go get lunch with a cousin and make them order the food for us. I would sidle into shops in the local mall, browse the aisles quickly with one eye glued on the nearest staff member, then scuttle back out again the moment they noticed me. Or, more commonly, I would go into a bookstore, find a quiet row of shelves at the back and flip through hundreds of paperbacks for an hour. Because that seemed to be the only place where customers could exist without being disturbed all the time.

I think my grandfather picked up on this aversion of mine. Guests would come round to his huge sprawling house to meet the British relatives and I would be shy and uncommunicative, giving short answers to every question and looking for the first chance to escape upstairs and lie down on a bed with a book. Surprisingly, he wasn't an overly talkative man himself. But he was a big community figure and among fellow farmers in a small rural town, social ties mean everything. He used to put an oversized General Motors baseball cap on my head and tell me to jump in his pickup truck because 'you and me are going down to see about The Bottoms'.

The Bottoms was his name for a large swathe of farmland, hidden way back from the road, where he'd spent a lifetime growing spinach. We'd pull off the highway and make our way down bumpy dirt roads, passing row after row — thousands, if not more — of uniformly planted crops. Then he'd slow down to a crawl and while his sun-beaten truck grumbled through miles of dust, he'd try to get me talking. Sometimes he told me stories from his childhood, like how he used to walk all the way to school in the Great Depression without any shoes on, and one time he'd stepped on a big iron nail that went straight through his foot. Other times he'd talk about the land and how to farm it. *When that spinach is ready, we harvest it fast. Doesn't matter if it's the middle of the night. We get everyone outta bed and they come on down here with spotlights.*

I tried to make the kind of conversation he wanted from me. But I could never come out with more than a polite British sentence or two. He was an imposing man, try as he might to put me at ease. And his world was alien to me. Even when he tried to steer things closer to home, asking me how I was doing at school or what my friends were like back in England, beyond giving him a quick, factual answer, I just didn't know what to say. It felt much more natural simply to listen. After a few of these drives, I think he kind of came to respect that. We'd lapse into mutual silence, looking out at dark green spinach fields quivering in the heat. All we could hear then was the low growl of his pickup, the endless croak of cicadas and the rhythmic hiss of irrigation pumps as they sprayed water across The Bottoms. In truth, I think we both felt more comfortable that way. Somehow the less we talked, the more it meant.

Meanwhile, after spending six weeks in Oklahoma for the entire summer holidays, there was always a new school term to come back home to. And when I was 10 years old, I returned to preparations for the Eleven Plus. This was the exam that all English children had to take before leaving primary school, to decide where their education would take them next. The test was designed to sort children into two camps: those with an aptitude for learning and those without it. In other words, the 'intelligent' and the 'unintelligent'. We understood the basic equation: do well in the Eleven Plus and you'll go to a good school, don't do well and you'll go to a bad school. Yet it meant so much more than that. It would ultimately decide who we'd grow up with, which universities we'd go to, which jobs we'd be eligible for, what kind of money we'd make, the sort of lives we'd come to lead. Go one step further and you might even call it a kind of social engineering.

As a result, parents got anxious about the future. They wanted the best for their kids, so they cranked up the pressure to maximise the chance of success. For the child, it was a lot of responsibility to shoulder at a young age: do not disappoint your parents and above all, do not let yourself down. The exam used to take place in the autumn. In the summer leading up to it, I was a bag of nerves.

My parents arranged for a private tutor to come to our house once a week and prepare me for the kind of questions I'd soon be facing. They were markedly different to the things we'd learnt so far in school and included verbal reasoning that supposedly indicated your IQ. Questions like this: 'PS is to RY as HL is to...<insert answer here>'. I would sit at the dining room table with my tutor, a retired teacher called Mrs Bonney who was friendly but business-like, and perform mock examinations to get me ready for the real thing.

The work was hard enough, because my primary school hadn't taught me to think in this way before (how did children without tutors stand a chance?). But what really troubled me was the setup of those practice exams. Mrs Bonney would sit down next to me, give me a dummy exam paper and start a stop-clock. I would then have 45 minutes to complete all the questions, while she watched over my shoulder and corrected or commended as I went.

And I found that intolerable. The room would fall silent, apart from the loud ticking of an old clock hung above our piano, and all I could think about was a pair of critical eyes watching my every move. By this time I was acutely conscious of the strange way I held my pen. For reasons I've never been able to pin down, all through primary school, I'd refused to write like everyone else. The rest of the children had adopted the 'tripod' grip, with the pen or pencil pinched between their first two fingers and thumb. But I gripped my pen in the way that felt most comfortable — by closing my hand into a fist. My teachers gave me a special triangular 'corrector' grip for my pen, to encourage me to put my fingers in the right place. But sooner or later I always took it off and went back to the bunched fist.

Mrs Bonney commented on it. And every time I sat before her in the dining room, with every mark I made on the page, I thought about how I couldn't write properly and how unimpressed she must have been. While she observed me at close quarters, my hands would start to sweat and leave wet marks on the exam booklet. As my tightly clenched fist worked its way down the questions, the margin of the page would grow damp and curl back on itself. I would press so hard with my pen that the next pages would have my answers carbon-copied onto them. I obsessed over these uncontrollable details instead of concentrating on my work.

This peaked, one time, when I was halfway through a mock paper. My bladder had been steadily swelling since Mrs Bonney had arrived but I'd hesitated, at the start, to ask if I could go to the bathroom. Now the stop-clock was running and I felt like it was too late. I couldn't interrupt the Fake Eleven Plus and, anyway, I was too embarrassed and self-conscious to bring it up. I convinced myself I could last until the session was over. But I was dead wrong. After a while, I reached the point of no return and I quietly wet myself right there in my seat. The hot urine soaked through my trousers and into the cushion on my dining-room chair. I waited, mortified, to see what my tutor would say. But she didn't seem to notice. And didn't say anything.

The exam ended before I could finish it and my answers were a lot worse than usual. Mrs Bonney frowned down at my scribbles and said with some puzzlement: 'something was distracting you today'. Had she really not noticed the dark stain running all the way down my legs? She seemed oblivious but was probably just sparing my feelings. Either way, her statement was so right but at the same time so wrong. Yes, something had definitely distracted me that day. But something distracted me every day, whether she was there or not. I was distracted by a gnawing fear of social contact. And I was already developing a fear of that fear. The vicious cycle was growing more defined and the only time it faded away into the background was when I could be by myself.

Just like my piano teacher, I believe my tutor thought I had some learning difficulties. We continued with our lessons and I continued to give mediocre results. How could I explain to them, or even to myself, that it wasn't the work itself that held me back? It was the beginnings of social anxiety.

In the end I passed the Eleven Plus by a few marks. It felt like a lead weight had been lifted off my back. I remember a happy few final terms at primary school. I'd secured a place at the local grammar school and my parents were very pleased. That relief wore off as I approached my first day at a new school.

# 11: House rules

Secondary school, from age 11 to 16, threw me into a whole new system. There were four houses at my new school — Blue, Brown, Green, Red. And I became a member of Red House. A healthy rivalry was promoted between houses and this was my first taste of tribal loyalties.

All boys stuck to their houses with a clear sense of us and them, so the first half of school wasn't the social nightmare I had feared because there was some safety in numbers. Everyone, by the nature of school, was finding their feet and making mistakes. We were exploring a new world in pre-assigned groups and for the next five years, in many ways, my confidence actually grew. I regularly spoke up in class and liked to get into debates with my teachers, particularly about ethics or religion. Because there were so many of us, it was easy to fade into the background. This was especially true of sports.

In the lower school, sports were mandatory but I only remember playing basketball, cricket and rugby, and only every once in a while, because my PE teachers were focused on creating young footballers. If you weren't interested in football, they weren't interested in you. Which was OK with me. As I'd already discovered with swimming, the expectation attached to sport was best avoided. Miss the goal and the other players jeered at you. Fumble a catch and your whole team paid the price. So, over the course of six years, I slowly but surely fell off the athletic radar, participating when I had to but always half-heartedly and always looking for ways to dodge a games lesson.

My favourite way to do this was during cross-country running. I really hated that miserable outdoors sport, which always happened in midwinter in overgrown fields full of waterlogged grass. It was cold, wet and muddy, but long stretches of those runs were unsupervised. At the first opportunity, after dropping behind the main pack, I'd cut behind a hedge and pull out a packet of Marlboro Lights, smoking two or three in quick succession, enjoying the nicotine head-rush and savouring the sense of an illicit crime. A rebellious moment, stolen from the powers that be.

I first tried smoking when I was about 13 and cigarettes quickly became a staple of my teenage years. Partly because I easily bent to peer pressure and whenever other people smoked, I did too. But also because it was a de facto mode of escape. Smoking had to be done in secret and in small groups, to avoid detection. We would disappear up to the top of our local park, where a ring of bushes hid us from view. Smoking was a solitary act, too. And perhaps that's why it appealed to me. I often went up to the roof of a multi-storey car park on my own, to smoke fags and watch the people going about their business way down below, oblivious to my existence.

Had I given it some thought I might have realised that smoking wasn't really an escape route. Long-term, it was more of a dead-end. As a stimulant, tobacco made my heart race and my thoughts soar – bad news for a growing case of social anxiety. It became something else I had to conceal, something else to be nervous about. I would come home from school with my uniform stinking of smoke, bypass my parents as fast as I could and run upstairs to spray Lynx deodorant all over myself. Then I'd scrub my fingers with soap and brush my teeth so hard that my gums bled. Even then I'd spend all my time worrying that it could be smelled. It was something I had to hide from other people's parents, too. I remember being at a friend's house once and while I was sitting on the sofa, my lighter somehow slipped out of my pocket and fell down between some cushions. Later on, when my friend's dad was on the sofa sitting in the exact same spot, he found the lighter, held it up and asked the room aloud:

'Oh yeah? Who's been on the fags, then?'

I went bright red and didn't know where to look. My friend's dad latched on to my reaction and made the most of it.

'You could light a cigarette off Russell's face right now.'

Looking back, was that a fair thing to say to a 13-year-old? He was chastising me, no doubt. Embarrassing me to make me think twice about smoking. But wasn't the blush enough? Why were some grown-ups so quick to call out my blushing, like they were getting a kick out of it? By this age I was already aware that I couldn't hide my emotions. If I had something to conceal, blushing would give it away. A sense of powerlessness started to creep up inside me.

At school, I saw other people who were powerless in other ways. I was never bullied at my single-sex school and I consider myself lucky. Because other boys weren't so lucky. One of my big regrets from this time is that I saw bullying and let it happen. Much to my shame, I sometimes joined in myself. Because I wanted to keep the spotlight off me.

There was one boy who was overweight and wore thick spectacles. He had wild, unwashed hair that never got cut and spoke in strange metaphors, quoting literature we hadn't read or scientific laws we didn't understand. He was fiercely intelligent and well ahead of his time. But to us he was just a weirdo. He was socially awkward and no one could relate to him. So he was mercilessly bullied all through school, just for being different. We hated people who didn't fit into our tribes. And he was in a different house, anyway. So he didn't matter to us one bit. He was marginalised until he disappeared without a trace after our GCSEs, leaving school to do — what, I wonder? How did he fare in the big wide world as an adult, after such horrible treatment as a boy?

I remember one time when the boys in Red House were in the middle of a lesson. There was a knock on the door and a boy from Blue House entered. Let's call him 'C'. C had been sent from another classroom with a message to give to our teacher. He was called into the room and asked what he wanted. C stood still in front of the chalkboard, wringing his hands and pursing his lips. His eyes darted back and forth from the teacher to the floor, then started bulging in his head as his cheeks puffed out. It looked like he was holding a ping pong ball inside his mouth, trying unsuccessfully to blow it out. The class quickly became aware of this strange behaviour and our natural instinct was to laugh at it. Somebody shouted out: 'just fucking say it'. I think I yelled: 'come on, spit it out'. Another person declared exactly what everyone else was thinking: 'oi, what's your problem?'. With the whole room ridiculing him, C's face continued to contort until our teacher escorted him into the hallway. A few minutes later, our teacher came back without C and gave us all a dressing down. That boy, she told us, had a stammer. And the way we'd treated him was unforgivable.

We hadn't known he stuttered. In truth, I don't think a lot of us really knew what a stutter was. But now that we did know, it became a fresh box of ammo that everyone used against him. He was taunted all through school for it. I can't remember if our teachers ever caught wind of this, but nobody ever seemed to come to his aid.

I find myself returning to that memory and putting myself in that boy's shoes. Sometimes, a single experience can help colour the rest of your life. Stuttering works in exactly the same way as blushing. The anticipation of humiliation leads to fear of the event; the humiliation during the event fuels further fear of it; the event then becomes something you'll do almost anything to avoid. Stuttering is involuntary and, although there are methods to treat it, I imagine it never fully goes away. You're born with it and it lurks like a shadow in the grey matter of your brain. That boy left school and became a man and his stutter probably stayed with him. I imagine it made him speak less, as a general rule, in favour of thinking more. It may have steered him into a career in the background. People may have mistaken his quietness for aloofness. Perhaps they judged him to be unfriendly. Over time, perhaps his circle of influence shrank smaller and smaller. Fewer acquaintances. Fewer friends. Fewer opportunities to meet the opposite sex. Speech impediments are known for decreasing a person's quality of life. They can limit who you are and who you will be. I'm willing to bet that C remembers that moment when he came into our classroom and his weakness was laid bare for all to see. I felt bad for him at the time. And yet I plunged the knife in just like everyone else.

Another pervading memory was the omnipresent fear of exams. We love exams in Britain. They help us draw a clearly defined line between success and failure, between those who can and those who can't. It's the beginnings of our class system, ingrained from an early age. What began with the Eleven Plus continued all through my secondary education at the end of every school year, when all students had to sit their end-of-term exams. They were the high point you aimed for throughout the academic year. And for many students, they were very much the low point.

Because your performance at the end of each year determined which 'stream' you entered in the next. Do badly in your maths exam, for example, and you were sent straight to the bottom stream to learn at a slower pace on simpler topics. And that's exactly what happened to me. I always struggled with numbers. That part of my brain just didn't work. I still struggle with numbers today, particularly mental arithmetic, when I find myself counting on my fingers or whispering aloud as I try to calculate in my head. So I ended up right at the bottom of the Maths pile. Where I was taught slowly and painstakingly.

English was a different story. I found reading and writing so much easier. For all other subjects — History, Geography, French, German, Biology, Chemistry, Physics — I was somewhere in between.

Regardless of how good you were at any subject, every year without fail, judgement day would come.

Our world revolved around this fixed point in the year. It hung over our heads, like an axe suspended up high, waiting to fall just before every summer holiday. For me, that moment always coincided with hayfever season. In late May or early June, I get extreme hayfever. Forget about itchy eyes and a scratchy throat, my immune system goes into revolt and my sinuses swell until they completely block my nose. For three or four weeks I can only breathe through my mouth. Nowadays it's an inconvenience. Back then, it felt like a very personal curse. Hayfever is classed as Hypersensitivity Type 1 (there are 5 types in total). It's becoming fashionable these days to suggest that introverts and shy people are genetically predisposed to sensitivity. On the physical side, they're more susceptible to allergies. On the emotional side, they're easily overwhelmed. Perhaps there's some truth in that. All I know is that heightened nervousness mixed with hayfever used to make me feel like I was under siege, inside and out. I felt entirely out of control.

I think that feeling drip-fed into what was becoming social anxiety. Exams were an early manifestation of that black zeppelin I described earlier: looming on the horizon, drifting closer with every passing day. An exam is a fixed point in the future you're afraid of. It's something to think about and stew about and slowly blow out of all proportion. As its shadow grows larger, it becomes another bad experience you wish you could avoid.

When the big day finally arrived, I would barely get any sleep the night before. I would wake up, shower and dress in a daze, then force myself to eat a bowl of cereal while feeling sick and nauseous in the pit of my stomach. Then I'd make the long slow march to school, my bag on my shoulder feeling like an iron weight dragging me down into the ground. My mouth dry and metallic. My palms clammy and wet.

Exams took place in the main assembly hall with scores of wooden desks lined up in rows. As we all worked on our papers in total silence, teachers would patrol the ranks to hand out spare pens and sheets of paper and check no one was cheating. The hours spent in an exam were a kind of depersonalisation, a sense of stepping outside yourself, of watching from a neutral distance. I remember nothing of the exam papers themselves. But I do recall vividly the woody smell of the parquet floors and the panelled walls in the main hall, the way motes of dust danced through shafts of sunshine coming in through the windows. And a lone shuttlecock that sat trapped inside an old air vent in the centre of the high ceiling. I would look around at these things, slowly observing the details, while my 'other' self agonised over the pages of my exam. It's always been that way for me: in moments of prolonged stress or panic, the big things would fade out and the small things would fade in.

After burning so much nervous energy in an exam, I'd feel depleted. There'd be a distant ring in my ears. My skin would tingle and prickle like pins and needles. I'd want nothing more than to go straight back home and lie down quietly.

I'm 40-plus years old now but I still get anxiety dreams about my school exams. In these semi-nightmares, I find myself getting lost while walking to school to sit a big exam. With every turn I take I get more and more lost. In my dream, it's still the mid-nineties and people don't have mobile phones. There's no way to call the school and tell them I'm late. All I can think about is how disappointed my parents will be. How angry my teachers will be and how much trouble I'm in. Sometimes, this is the last exam left until I'm free from school forever. But obstacle after obstacle stands between me and it. And it's all my own fault. I've failed everybody who ever cared about me and worst of all, I've failed myself...

Then I wake up, sweating all over. It takes me a few bewildered seconds to realise I'm not a schoolboy anymore. And a profound sense of gratitude seeps in.

It's a powerful myth that's taken root in my subconscious. Much like SAD, it's an involuntary part of my psyche and if I had a choice, I'd remove it. But I can't. It lives there permanently, planted long ago. We put a lot of pressure on kids in the UK, at a very young age. I can't help but think it has implications for our mental health later on.

# 12. The Sixth Form

Very suddenly, at the age of 16, it was time to reshuffle the pack. More than half the kids I'd grown up with for the last five years failed their GCSE exams, meaning they couldn't come back to join the Sixth Form after the summer holidays. They went out into the real world to try and find jobs or enrol at a different college to take their studies further. For about a year I saw some familiar faces hanging around the high street or kicking a ball in the local parks. But I never saw most of those boys again.

Those of us who did come back were immediately aware of a sense of social sorting. Houses didn't mean anything, anymore. There were no more packs to hide in. Instead, a big emphasis was placed on the individual. We stopped wearing identical uniforms. Instead we were allowed to wear our own suit and tie. Your life from this point was up to you. You had to believe in yourself and your future career. You were a Sixth Former, now, and your destiny was up to you. There was a lot of talk like that in assemblies and lessons, in the first few weeks. And the level of expectation made me feel uncomfortable from day one.

Everything I've ever read about social anxiety in books and online suggests that SAD arrives with a bang in early adolescence, when kids are in their late teens. I was a textbook example of this. All of a sudden, as though someone had pressed a neurological button, I couldn't stand being in close proximity to other people. Everything in this changed school environment revolved around social skills. There was no more 'Sir' or 'Miss'. Now, our teachers encouraged us to address them by name and talk to them on their level. We were told to engage with our peers as fellow adults. We had group discussions, formal presentations, open debates — full of the topics and techniques that would make us successful young men at university and beyond. I hated any moment that forced me to make myself known to others.

I was blushing a lot, by now. At anything and everything. I would blush if someone started a conversation with me or, very often, before they even came over to start it. I would blush deeply as I entered a room, whether people were looking at me or not. Other boys picked up quickly on it. How could they not? It then became a daily, if not an hourly, struggle. My world divided into two camps:

those who made fun of me when I blushed and those who didn't. Those who did were endlessly following the same routine.

'Why have you gone so red?'

I would have no answer for this. So they would stand there, staring at me, forcing me to give them a reply.

'I don't know. I'm just hot.'

'But your face is always red. Are you always hot?'

'I don't know.'

'Look at him. He's gone even redder!'

I remember one time, I was in a shop buying my lunch when a boy I knew from school marched up to me from nowhere. He was a cocky kid, always outspoken and always looking for ways to start trouble. He had two pretty girls with him and a big grin plastered across his face. He stopped me dead in my tracks, looked me in the eye and said:

'Alright Russell? I want you to say hello to Jessie and Sarah.'

Automatically, because I'd been pulled into a conversation unprepared and three people were now staring at me – two of them attractive young women – my face flooded with blood. I stood there, trying to ignore my burning face while I answered.

'How's it going?'

But they didn't answer me back. The boy looked at the girls, who started giggling. One of them pulled a camera out of her pocket and snapped a photo of me. The boy burst out laughing and led them both away. 'See? I told you. So fucking awkward!'

I always wondered why those girls were so keen to humiliate a total stranger. I'd never seen them before. But I did see them again, about a year later, at a house party. Where they reminded me about 'that time you went so red'. And tried to make me do it again.

I don't class that kind of behaviour as bullying. Everyone got teased at my school, to one extent or another. At no time was I physically hurt. I was never forced into a fight after school while dozens of other kids watched and cheered, like some of the other boys I knew. I was never systematically targeted, even if perhaps it felt that way sometimes. Of the boys who'd made it through to the Sixth Form, I still had a small but close group of friends from Red House. Unlike some of the newcomers who joined us from other schools who spent two years trying to infiltrate closed-off groups, I was never truly alone amidst 100-odd bored, immature, adolescent young men.

And bored is the crucial word. As we made our way through the last two years of school, our learning intensified but it also slowed down to a snail's pace. Now that everyone had narrowed their studies down to three or four subjects, we all had different timetables. And those timetables were full of 'free periods' scattered across the week. We were supposed to use those hours for extra study in our common room or in the school library. But realistically this free time just meant that boys would aimlessly congregate in the nearest empty classroom, keen to mess about. When a teacher passed, everyone would pretend to read or get on with some work. And as soon as the coast was clear, it was straight back to banter and play-fights.

I found all that spare time close to unbearable. Being trapped in a room with restless boys often felt like an experience that had no end. The way we harassed each other physically and mentally, minute after minute, hour after hour, slowly made me a nervous wreck. I was always waiting for the focus to fall on me, for everyone to start making fun of my bashfulness. On bad days, I would gradually sink into a Slow Blush – going redder and redder, wanting so badly to get away from everyone and just be by myself. I would look up at the clock and watch the second hand crawling around the dial, praying for it to move quicker and bring me closer to my next lesson. To some kind of distraction, some kind of order.

So I fell into the habit of hiding whenever a free period was coming up. We had an old communal toilet block at my school, a long brick building with rows of toilet cubicles and sinks inside. I used to hide in a cubicle for an hour, terrified every time I heard the main door burst open and a group of boys come tumbling inside. When I wasn't employing that tactic, I would get an exeat – a slip of paper giving me permission to spend some time off the school premises – and go to the bigger library in the town centre. It was easy to get lost in there. I'd find a study booth tucked away in a corner and soak up the solitude, surrounded by the deep silence found only in libraries. And the comforting papery smell of hundreds and hundreds of books. After a while, some of my closer friends learnt my habits. When I disappeared from school, they came looking for me in the toilets or hunted me down in the town library. I hated it when they discovered me, because although they were my pals and I liked them a lot, I still felt on edge in their presence. Especially when they'd caught me in the act, hiding away from them. Why was I running away from people? Especially those people I called friends? I was painfully aware that I must have seemed odd to everyone.

Time wore on and it got to the point where I wanted to avoid school altogether. On days when I had lots of anxious free periods lined up, I would get up in the morning, get dressed, eat breakfast and leave the house as normal around 8am. By then, my dad would have driven off to London. He wouldn't be back until the evening. My mum didn't leave for her job at a local school until 10am. It meant that, whenever I had no intention of going to school, I had two hours ahead of me I needed to kill. I couldn't go towards the town centre or someone from school might see me. I couldn't stay too close to home or I might run into someone my parents knew. So I used to walk just far enough away from my house to feel safe. I'd wander through suburban backstreets for half a mile or so. Then I'd pick three or four roads that felt quiet and empty – and start walking around them in circuits. I had nothing to do and nowhere to go. I would walk in circles past the same flats and houses again and again, trying not to look suspicious. I winced every time a car drove past, worried it would slow down and a teacher or a neighbour would get out to ask me what I was doing here. I would try to find quiet places every now and then to smoke a cigarette, maybe a row of garages behind some flats or an alleyway that cut between houses. Staying still for long felt too dangerous. So I always tried to keep moving.

As I trudged up and down residential streets, feeling isolated and paranoid, I remember asking myself: why am I like this? Am I mentally ill? Something wasn't right. But anything was preferable to spending the day in discomfort at school.

Eventually, 10am would roll around. I'd slowly make my way back to my house with its now-empty driveway. Mum was gone, the coast was clear and I could take cover indoors until she came back at 5pm, when I'd pretend I'd just come in from school. I'd spend the day reading books and watching classic movies on TV. I'd make myself a huge sandwich for lunch then sit in the garden, if the sun was out, listening to the unmistakable sound of wood pigeons. What began as a morning filled with fear quickly became an afternoon of relief. Those hours spent on my own were nourishing in ways I didn't understand. I needed them badly but I didn't know why. All I knew for sure was that I'd get in trouble for this, sooner or later. I could only sustain it for so long. But while it lasted, on and off for almost a year and a half, the peace it gave me made the risk feel worth it.

Back in the Sixth Form, my responsibilities were increasing. As we progressed to the Upper Sixth, my deputy headmaster wanted to turn us all into Prefects. At first he asked for volunteers. Then he started choosing people at random. Eventually, it started to feel like a military draft. Everyone had to sign up at some point and it was only a matter of time until your name was next on the list. Being a Prefect was something I needed to avoid at all costs. It would mean doing things that were unthinkable; like getting up on-stage to give a speech or say a prayer during assemblies or – even worse – being put in charge of a whole class of younger boys. Prefects had to monitor younger kids during detentions or keep them in check whenever teachers weren't around. You were expected to show confidence and leadership so the younger kids would respect you. But in reality it just meant they were always looking for weaknesses. If you showed even a sliver of self-doubt, they would tear you apart. Being a Prefect would be utterly impossible and I worked hard to make myself scarce whenever the possibility arose. By the time I left school, I was one of about 10 boys who'd managed to avoid becoming a Prefect. At the time I felt like I'd enjoyed a lucky escape.

Now, I just feel sad for my younger self. Because I've learnt that accepting a challenge, even one you're likely to fail, makes you a stronger person. Being a Prefect would have forced me to take a step forward, instead of always taking a step back. But how could I possibly have explained that to my 18-year-old self?

Back then I was studying English Lit, English Language and Art. Each of these subjects gave me new things to dread. In English Lit, we made our way through classics like Hamlet and Dr Faustus by taking on the role of a character and reading their lines out loud during lessons. I never raised my hand to participate. In English Language, we had to work on our own projects and present them back to the class. The presenter was chosen at random, so I found myself living on tenterhooks, week in week out, fearing the moment when my name would get called out and I'd have to stand up and go red and sweaty and have a very public meltdown in front of my peers. Art was definitely easier. I spent a lot of time blending paints behind an easel or sketching quietly with charcoal. But there were still times when I had to show my work and talk through it with my teacher. I was self-conscious of my creations and excruciatingly self-conscious when I had to speak up for them.

As I'd expected, my school absences caught up with me in the end. As the Sixth Form was finishing and our A-Levels were about to begin, we had a parents' evening. My mum and dad found out about the lessons I'd been missing. It meant my predicted grades were lower than expected, which would affect the universities I could apply to. My teachers were mostly of the opinion I was unengaged and withdrawn, generally quite able but lacking motivation and will. I remember keenly, at that time, wondering why nobody suspected anything else. My teachers believed I was slacking off. And my dad certainly believed the same. After that meeting, he put me under house arrest with strict orders to 'pull a miracle out of my arse' and pass my final exams.

How could I say to my teachers, to my parents: I don't come to school because being around people fills me with panic? The reality of social anxiety, especially when you're still a child, is that you simply don't understand it. You can't explain it to yourself, let alone the people who are mistaking it for something else. So I went along with the narrative that I'd stopped caring, that my skills were coming up short. Even though, in my own head, I knew the opposite was true. I may have been skipping school but I was still keeping up with my studies. I knew my subjects inside out and had confidence in my knowledge. Especially when it came to answering exam questions in the way examiners liked.

But my Art exam was scheduled to last for three days, in a room full of boys. On the morning of day two, I needed to go out to a DIY shop to buy a pot of glossy black paint. I left the school grounds and bought the paint but the thought of returning to a packed classroom was too much for me. I've always found it hard to go into a room when I know people are inside it and all eyes will turn to me as soon as I appear through the door. So I hid in an alleyway behind the DIY shop for a few hours, until lunchtime, so I could slip back into the Art room unnoticed. I remember my teacher asking me where I'd been with an incredulous look in his eyes. It was just one more reason to think I wasn't taking my studies seriously.

When our results finally came through, I'd passed everything. I got an A in English Lit, an A in English Language and a B in Art. I felt vindicated, to a certain degree, as though I'd proved the point that what you see isn't always what you get. My parents were happy, my teachers were happy. But I spent the rest of that summer mostly unhappy, after taking a job in the pot wash of a local French restaurant. I disappeared for seven days a week into a hot, cramped back-room, scrubbing pots, pans, dishes and knives from lunchtime through till dinner. I was literally hiding in there, not even coming out to eat a free lunch with the rest of the staff because I was too scared to sit at a table and eat with them, in case I blushed. There were times when the restaurant was short on staff, so I had to serve front-of-house as a waiter. I absolutely hated it. I was racked with nerves when taking orders and dealing with customers.

A few months later I got confirmation that I'd been accepted to the University of Birmingham. I chose Birmingham for two reasons. First, it was the only uni that would let me study Archaeology (my new-found interest) alongside English. And second, it was where my older sister had gone. Beyond that, there was no other reason why I chose the Midlands. But that's where I was headed for the next three years.

# 13. Bad rituals

University didn't start well for me. I almost got kicked out on day one.

When I arrived in Birmingham I went straight to my student halls, an old converted mansion called Manor House where Lord Cadbury (of milk chocolate fame) used to live. I was anxious about living with complete strangers and all the weeks of 'getting to know you' that were coming my way. So I overcompensated for my lack of confidence and went completely the other way.

On our first night there, after many welcome drinks, a party started that grew out of control. It was like something you'd see in a US frat house: toilet rolls being thrown up into trees, eggs being thrown down at people from open windows. I really can't think why I'd brought it with me but I owned, at that time, a small air gun and several boxes full of plastic pellets. It was a realistic-looking gun, a model of a black Beretta pistol. When I was suitably drunk and the party was suitably wild, I went to my new bedroom and unpacked the gun. I loaded it with pellets and went to the third floor of my block. There was a breakaway party happening up there in someone else's dorm room. I passed the gun around and a few people (i.e. all the males in the room) wanted to see it in action. So I opened up a window that looked down onto a grassy courtyard outside, where dozens of freshers were shouting and mucking about in drunken groups. And I started shooting people in the crowd. At random. While the whole room behind me cheered and laughed.

I do wonder at my complete ignorance back then. To me this was no big deal. It was an air gun, a plastic toy. I was joining in the fun and games and I had a drunken desire to impress people. At no point did it cross my mind that I was in the middle of a student residence, leaning out of a window, waving around a large replica handgun.

Someone called up the Manor House Dean and told him a student was threatening people from a top-floor window with a gun. Within minutes the party got shut down. Wardens turned up with flashlights, everyone was ordered inside and the students out in the courtyard were taken away to be questioned. It wouldn't be long at all before I was identified as the culprit but I remained totally oblivious. I went back to my room and put the gun under some socks in a drawer, thinking that was the end of it. But then the Dean and two wardens knocked on my door and asked for permission to search my room. In a panic, I said yes. And the Dean diligently worked his way through all my possessions. He found the gun and the ammo soon enough, confiscated everything and told me to wait for further instructions tomorrow.

To cut a long story short, I went through the university's disciplinary procedure, involving a mock court hearing with eyewitnesses and a panel of judges. The seriousness of the situation, which I still hadn't grasped, was finally hammered home. Aside from the danger imposed on other students (they told me someone could have been blinded — and they were right) there was the danger I'd put the university's reputation in. They didn't want stories like this in the press and they didn't want loose cannons like me running around Manor House causing trouble. But it was my first week in Birmingham and everyone agreed to take this into account. So instead of expelling me and killing my degree before it started, they gave me the maximum fine of £200 (a lot of money when I was 19) and a warning to be on my best behaviour from now on at all times.

Was I a loose cannon? I was deeply embarrassed by the whole thing. Sitting there in a chair while a roomful of people interrogated me was agony. It was bad enough to feel ashamed already but sitting in the spotlight with so many eyes burning into me was, albeit unknown to them, a very personal torture. In an effort to make a bold first impression, I'd behaved out of character. Now I just wanted to creep back inside my shell. I felt like persona non grata around Manor House after that. I was known as the guy who'd shot a bunch of people and got caught. It gave me a level of attention I didn't really want.

Living in halls was something of a shock to the system. Men and women stayed on separate floors, with single-sex toilets and showers, which wasn't so different from school. But everything else was communal, including meal times. To get your breakfast and dinner you had to queue up outside the dining hall. This queue would wind all the way round the corridor and once you joined it, you were stuck there for 20 minutes or more, talking to whoever you'd ended up next to. Twice daily I had that familiar sense of being trapped. Quite literally trapped in a narrow space, being forced to interact. I would sweat and blush and shift nervously from one foot to another, desperately willing the line to move quicker as it inched towards the dining hall door. Then, once inside with my tray full of food, I'd sit down at a communal table and go through the whole thing again, caught in a group of people, some I knew and some I didn't, chewing my food without enjoyment all tense and on-edge, watching the clock tick slower and slower on the dining room wall.

We had a student bar in the Manor House. A single carpeted room with about a dozen tables. It was the only place I felt comfortable because the lights were low in there and I could always have a pint of beer in my hand. Throughout my first year, I was in that bar every night of the week. I was over 18 now and a legal drinker. I'd already discovered how helpful alcohol could be. I loved it when my inhibitions came down and my confidence went up. It was something of a magic ticket. All I had to do was drink the right amount and I could behave like a normal person, without feeling confined, without adrenaline pumping through my veins every time somebody looked at me or spoke to me.

The boys on my floor were drinkers too. They happily came to the bar every night and, as long as the beer was flowing, I enjoyed getting to know them. But I would just as happily have gone there alone, something I often did in many pubs around the Birmingham campus. I'd find a corner table and decamp there for the afternoon, reading a newspaper or a novel and slowly getting drunk.

I was studying English and Ancient History & Archaeology, with two very different crowds of students. I was equally terrified of each. Lectures weren't so bad. They were a one-way broadcast. You could sit in a sea of students and simply observe. I used to turn up for them at the last possible moment, so I wouldn't have to stand around with other people in the hallway outside. When the lesson was finished,

I would either leave the lecture hall immediately or hang back until the room had emptied, then make my escape without speaking to anyone. Over that first year I made very few friends, on either side of my degree. In fact the only people I really got to know, for my full three years at Birmingham, would be the boys I first drank with back in my halls.

Along with lectures came the more intimate setting of seminars. And they rapidly became a problem. In those smaller and more interactive learning groups, there really was no place to hide. They came around once a week or so and I dreaded being in a room with five or six people, arranged in a circle, expected to openly debate a book or journal.

So I developed a bad ritual. An hour or so before every seminar, I disappeared into the library to find a solo study booth. There were lots of them dotted around, tucked away in nooks and crannies between vast and dusty rows of books. These booths were designed so that one person could vanish from the rest of the world and immerse themselves in their work.

But I had a different kind of immersion in mind. In my bag would be a newly bought bottle of alcohol. For some reason, at that point in life, it was always cheap white vermouth. Probably because it packed more punch than wine but wasn't as expensive as a spirit. I would leisurely drink from the bottle, pacing each mouthful over the next hour so I'd polish the whole thing off about five minutes before the seminar began. Then, my mouth hot and tingling with dry and bitter herbs, I'd hurry across the campus to the Humanities block and walk into the seminar – pleasantly drunk.

For the next hour, I'd talk much more than usual. All the things I wanted to say about the poetry we were reading or the ancient plays we were studying, but was normally too afraid to share, came out with ease. I was playing my part as an engaged student and felt good about it. Everyone else in the room must have noticed the difference, though. Looking back, it was so obvious. I must have reeked of booze. Quickly brushing my teeth or sucking a mint beforehand never occurred to me, I just went straight into those sessions with a brain full of fortified wine. Surely it showed in my eyes, my voice. But no one ever said anything, at least not to my face. My tutors noticed nothing at all. They just seemed pleased I was contributing to the group. For a brief hour I felt empowered to be myself.

It quickly waned, of course. By the end of the seminar I was already starting to come down. My eyes had grown heavy, my mouth had gone dry. Drinking a whole bottle like that in the middle of the day would wreck my whole afternoon. I'd slump back to Manor House and fall into bed, sleep heavily until the evening and wouldn't be able to get back to sleep that night. I'd lie in bed until the early hours, feeling like a total failure. Why couldn't I do the most basic things... sit with people, talk to people... without downing a bottle of booze first?

This behaviour carried on for about six months. After that, I vowed to break the cycle and stop. Which meant a return to 60-minute seminars full of sweating and mumbling and blushing: a weekly death by a thousand cuts. I feared that so much that I stopped going to seminars altogether. The first few times, I explained it away with illness. I used to drop notes into my tutors' pigeon-holes, telling them there'd been a sudden illness in my family. *Apologies but I've had to go back to London at very short notice. Please find my latest essay enclosed. I hope to see you next week but unfortunately I can't say if I'll be there for sure.* I used to say to myself 'next week will be better, I'll stop being so pathetic and I'll go'. But when the time came, it was just easier to avoid it. I did this for two whole semesters, completing the required work while being wholly absent. The students in my study group remained complete strangers. I had never even met some of my tutors. I felt bad about pretending my family was ill, what if I tempted fate and something terrible really did happen? But the guilt didn't outweigh the fear. This was textbook social anxiety, feeding itself like a virus. The more opportunities you miss, the more ways you will find to keep on missing them.

I'd fallen into bad rituals with the opposite sex, too. Coming of age in an all-boys school meant I knew nothing whatsoever about women. I couldn't talk to a woman or look her in the eye without blushing deeper and deeper shades of red. I couldn't make simple conversation. I didn't know what to do or when to do it. And so, on the very few occasions I did manage to get friendly with a girl, they would feel like rare victories over my social anxiety. I would overcompensate, just like I had with the air gun, by pouring myself too keenly into the situation.

And so a pattern would form. I'd get close to a girl who liked talking to me. We would quickly become confidantes. I would fall almost immediately in love, smitten with someone who was willing to look past my constant nerves and awkwardness. But I would keep it hidden for the longest possible time. When my feelings were eventually revealed, always far too late, they weren't reciprocated. But the friendship would continue anyway, with me hating myself because the whole thing now seemed dishonest but I was too scared to put a stop to it. There was a chance, perhaps, that things could still change? I lived in jaded hope like that, more than once, for relationships that were never going to happen.

Sooner or later these friendships ended in rejection. Something an all-male school definitely hadn't prepared me for. Rejection felt like failure on a primal level, more proof that there was something fundamentally wrong with me. So I stayed single throughout university while all around me, all the time, boys and girls were hooking up — seemingly without effort. In the end it made me question my sexuality. Maybe my failure with women was a sign and perhaps I'd have better luck with men? That's the path of reasoning social anxiety took me down next.

Lots of the artists I admired back then — musicians, painters, writers — were gay or bisexual. I was listening to lots of David Bowie and Lou Reed and Iggy Pop. The stories they told and the lives they'd led seemed so exciting to me. I wanted a taste of the freedom, the daring, the mysteriousness that seemed to come with a floating sexual identity. Of the small group of friends I'd made so far, almost all of them from my halls, more than a few were gay. So I started going to gay clubs with my gay friends. Sometimes I'd wear make-up like a glam rockstar. And in these unfamiliar places, I'd go about the business of being somebody else. Living an underground life was a thrill. For me, the gay nightlife seemed so illicit, so exotic, so other. Partly, perhaps, because lots of these bars were in nondescript warehouses or under railway arches in the old industrial hubs of Birmingham.

In reality, though, all I was doing was intruding in a space that wasn't illicit, exotic or other for any of the people who went there. The gay men and women in these clubs were just being themselves and no matter how hard I tried to fit in, everyone knew I was straight.

Who was I trying to kid? I wasn't homosexual. I was just desperate for love. So as quickly as that experiment started, it ended.

At the close of my first year, I failed some of my exams. I remember coming back to uni early after the summer holidays to resit the failed papers. I spent one happy week alone in my new accommodation, a three-storey house converted into student rooms, empty until the rest of my housemates showed up. I passed my exams this time and entered year two.

It was a year of hiding in plain sight. My anxiety took on a new facet and I developed a strong fear of being seen by people. In extreme cases, this is sometimes called *scopophobia*. I don't think my case was extreme. I didn't stay indoors for weeks on end to avoid the gaze of others, as true scopophobics will. But I did try to make myself as invisible as possible. I never took the bus to campus because the odds of seeing someone I knew and being trapped with them for the rest of the journey were high. Instead, I walked three miles to university every day, then three miles back again, to ensure I'd be alone the whole way. Every muscle would be poised for flight. If I saw anyone I knew in the distance, I'd quickly turn around and walk away in the other direction. Or I'd duck into the toilets or a nearby shop and wait 10 minutes until the coast was clear. I used to stay on the campus intentionally late, studying books and papers I didn't need to read, so I wouldn't have to go home and sit in the communal living room with my housemates.

I didn't want to prepare my food in their presence or eat it while they watched me, either. So I'd go to a kebab shop or a fish-and-chip place and eat my dinner on a plastic tabletop, watching the rain run grimly down the windows. Later in that second year, I spent three weeks abroad. The Archaeology Dept used to send students off on a Study Tour. You planned a mini thesis, went out to Greece or Italy or Spain and toured the ancient sites and ruins there to gather your evidence and prove your thesis. Most students paired off together or made small travelling teams so they could visit sites together. The idea of doing this terrified me, so I made a three-week itinerary that let me embark on my study tour alone. I was studying colonial Greek art and architecture, the temples and statues the Greeks built when they took over parts of Italy. I started in Rome, went down through Naples, down to Taranto, then across the sea to Sicily. And from there it was Siracusa, Gela and Palermo. In many ways it was three weeks of bliss; sun-soaked ruins, lots of time to write and reflect and wander around sleepy piazzas and flower-filled gardens. But at the same time it was very difficult. I couldn't speak a word of Italian. I was too timid to go into restaurants to eat food or ask people for help. I'd buy food and water from mini-markets where I could and pass through the checkout desk with nothing but cursory sign language. I'd sit on park benches to eat or make simple sandwiches back in my hotel room. I lost a lot of weight and started feeling weak towards the end of the trip.

Then, on my way back through Naples, I got mugged. I was struggling to find the train station when a smiling young teenager came over and struck up a conversation with me in broken English. He was friendly, he was good-looking (I still had a vague notion at that point that maybe I was gay) and he said he'd show me the quickest way to Napoli Centrale. It was just through these housing blocks, off the back of the Bay of Naples. We were halfway down some winding backstreets, laughing at our inability to communicate with each other, when he suddenly turned on me, all puffed up and violent. He threw me against a wall, pulled some loose change out of my pockets and ripped a gold chain my parents had given me off my neck. He hit me hard in the face a few times and then ran off.

Feeling numb, I found my way to the station and got onboard the first train leaving for Rome. When I got there, I found a telephone booth and phoned up my dad. When I spoke to him down the mouthpiece, my voice felt all crackly and dry. I told him I was back in Rome now and I'd just been robbed in Naples but everything was OK. He couldn't hear what I was saying and kept asking me to repeat it again. It wasn't because the connection was bad or because there were hundreds of cars and scooters grumbling past behind me. I realised my voice had almost disappeared because I hadn't used it for three weeks. I had to strain hard to make any sound come out at all. We take it for granted how often we use our voice. And don't realise how quickly it will go away if we don't.

I didn't get a good grade for my study tour. My tutor told me that, while it was bold to follow my own agenda and travel solo, I really should have teamed up with some other students to bounce my ideas off. My writing was too lofty and needed a strong argument to pin it down. Most people had co-written their theses and brought the best of two arguments together. Why hadn't I?

I knew the answer, but I had no reply. So I just sat on the other side of the desk, going slowly red, waiting for my first chance to end the conversation and escape from the room.

I went home that year sure that I was about to fail my degree.

# 14. Symptoms

In my third and final year, I moved into a small house much closer to the main campus. It was a dark and cramped little terrace, one of 200 identical homes lining the road from one end to the other. The sun never seemed to come in through the windows in that place. And the central heating didn't work. I lived with three other male students who I'd known since my first days in halls. I already knew I hated communal living but it was inside this house, with its tiny rooms and paper-thin plasterboard walls, that an overwhelming sense of claustrophobia took hold of me.

My workload was much heavier now. There were piles and piles of reading to be done for my English degree. And even more ancient texts to get through in Archaeology. The students I shared the house with were each in their final year of Music, Drama and Geography (respectively) and seemed to be loving every minute of it. I couldn't square their experience with mine. I was drowning in work and drawing further and further into myself. They were revelling in their studies and at the peak of their sociability. They'd bring girls home and have loud sex in their bedrooms. Or else they'd bring boys back to mess around with on the sofa late at night, just a few steps away from my door. My room was on the ground floor, a pokey little space just off the front hallway that once upon a time would have been a reception room. It was never meant to be a bedroom. The windows were single-glazed and looked straight out onto the street, so I kept the curtains drawn almost all day long. My housemates were constantly walking past my room as they went to and from the front door. I could hear everything that everyone said or did in the rest of the house. There was no escaping others.

So I spent almost all my time hidden away in my room, carefully avoiding the people I lived with. To get to the kitchen or bathroom, you had to get through the living room. And the living room was where my housemates spent most of their time. I'd listen carefully at my door and whenever the coast sounded clear, which really wasn't that often, I'd creep quickly into the kitchen to eat some toast or scoff down a sandwich. Or I'd strategically rush to the bathroom because I'd be bursting for the toilet. People were regularly in the living room for hours on end, so I fell into the awful habit of urinating into empty pint glasses that I kept in my room for that purpose. Then emptying them down the loo in the middle of the night. After a covert trip outside my room, I'd quickly rush back. And if I ran into anyone en route, I'd blush bright red and find the next few minutes of conversation excruciating. The others renting the house had known me for three years but they must have had some peculiar thoughts about me, by that point. The worst times were in the evenings, when they were all at home and cooking their dinners in the kitchen. Once they'd eaten, they'd sit in the lounge watching TV well into the night. And the whole time, I stayed secluded on my side of the door, wishing I was on another planet.

It was a slow, grey year and I passed almost all of it inside that room, only emerging for lectures or to go out and get smashed in the pubs. I developed a bad shaving rash that spread all over my face and chin, which just made me want to hide from public view even more. I became truly petrified of human contact. All my real friends (so I told myself) were studying in other cities far away from Birmingham. It was always raining. I couldn't get a girlfriend. I was going to fail my degree. I was going to have no career. How could working life after uni be anything but a car wreck if I was afraid of every person I met? I hated being alone but it was the only way I could function. And I couldn't even be alone with the door shut in my own bedroom. Everything converged and life lost its colour. Halfway through that last year something inside me, wearily treading water up until then, went still and started to sink.

I had never been depressed before. Or at least I don't think I had. My environment beforehand, living with my parents and spending every day at school, had somehow precluded it. Or perhaps depression arrives more commonly when you're a little older. Either way, I'd been completely independent and left to my own devices for almost three years now – and I'd grown sick of my own company. I knew the balance had tipped when I did something that had never crossed my mind before. I started to self-harm.

The first time I did it, I was in a nightclub. I'd gone out with a few people and we were all up on a stage, drunk and dancing in a crowd. I didn't want to be there and felt like a fraud, acting happy on the outside when I was despondent on the inside. Every time I thought no one was looking, I threw my fist angrily at the wooden wall next to me – disguising it like a dance move – punching it again and again, harder and harder, wanting to break my whole hand. Or snap a finger. I ended up doing neither and woke up the next morning with grazed knuckles and purple bruises. My body was a lot more resilient than I'd thought.

So I got more precise the next time and used a kitchen knife instead. I started with small, clean cuts on the back of my hands. The time after that, I worked my way up my forearms making long horizontal incisions. They were shallow cuts and they hurt, but they didn't bleed much. So the time after that, I cut deeper. I chose a meat knife with tiny serrations all along its edge, so it did its work more easily. My arm would trickle with blood for a bit while I dabbed it with tissues. But sometimes, when I pressed down harder, the knife would catch on a piece of muscle or fat and stop still. I'd have to pull it harder through my flesh, making a horrible little tearing noise. Strangely, most of those deeper cuts didn't bleed at all. And they took a lot longer to heal. I did this to myself a handful of times, always late at night, usually after drinking. And when I woke up in the morning I'd cover up the newly-formed scabs with plasters.

I remember keenly, one summer's day, when my dad and my nan came up to Birmingham to visit me. I'd been cutting my arms the night before. We went for a pub lunch and sat on a bench outside in the beer garden. I wore a long-sleeved shirt the whole time, to cover up the plasters criss-crossing my arms from the wrists to the elbows. I remember how hot the sun was, beating down on my shirt. How much my arms were itching and burning under the sleeves. And how ashamed I was to be sitting there, with two people who loved me dearly, with such a selfish secret.

If they only knew: all they had to do was pull up my sleeves and they'd see everything. They'd be so upset with me. My dad was funding my way through uni and this is how I repaid him? My nan had always believed in me and this is how I repaid her? I couldn't, at all costs, let them know how I really felt or what I was really doing to myself. So I just sat there and forced down a big lunch, chatting cheerfully, completely disgusted with myself.

It's going to be hard to explain the logic of self-harm. It's tempting to say there's no logic at all but there's a very definite path of internal reasoning your mind follows. 'Disgust with myself' was the endpoint I arrived at. It started simply with sadness. I was sad I couldn't fit in, sad I was always alone. Which made me feel powerless. My anxiety had all the power and I was powerless against it. Which made me feel worthless. And when you're worthless, it doesn't matter if you get damaged. In fact, you deserve pain and injury for being such a waste of space.

If I look closely at my arms now, 20 years later, I can still see thin white lines of scar tissue. And the sight of them makes me deeply embarrassed. (Thankfully, they've faded to a point that nobody notices them.) When I read back the thought process I've just described above, it sounds absurd to me. But at the time it consumed me and framed my whole personality. I was convinced of my own pointlessness. The scars on my skin remind me just how deeply I was deceiving myself and just how far anxiety had led me astray. I had no outside influences. I was stuck inside my own echo chamber. Self-harming was a new low for me. And even though, while doing it, I told myself it served me right – the next day, the sight of a dozen plasters in the mirror told me I'd taken a dreadfully wrong turn. I decided it was time to take a leap of faith instead and ask somebody for help.

That somebody was my family GP. On my next trip back home to London, I secretly booked an appointment with him. I was apprehensive: he was friends with my mum and dad, his son went to school with my younger brother, surely if I told him what was happening it would somehow come back to haunt me? I was vaguely aware of doctor/patient confidentiality and something called the Hippocratic Oath. But when I sat across from him inside his stuffy office, I could barely meet his eye. I told him I was finding my studies really hard. I was finding it even harder to socialise. He listened patiently, probing occasionally with carefully weighted questions.

Then it all came pouring out of me. I told him I felt miserable; I couldn't control my nerves and they had complete control of me; I was always hot and sweaty and always blushing at the slightest little thing; sometimes, it felt like my blood was on fire; I felt trapped and terrified when I had to spend time with other people; I avoided them at all costs because just being in their company filled me with horror and panic. Three years of worry and frustration all came out in one go and it was all I could do to stop myself from bursting into tears right there in the doctor's chair.

My GP stayed perfectly calm and scribbled down some notes. He said I was having a lot of intrusive thoughts. Did I ever act on those thoughts? I supposed the cuts on my arms were evidence of that. But I stopped short of revealing them. I said yes, I act on them, but I feel like they're acting on me and I'd give anything to stop them controlling every moment in my life. He tapped on his computer for a little bit, thinking. He asked me to take a blood test to see if I had an over-active thyroid. But in the meantime, here were two prescriptions: one for some medication that would lower my blood pressure and another for an antidepressant called Seroxat.

I saw the nurse before I left the surgery and she took a vial of my blood. Then I walked straight to the nearest pharmacist, feeling like I'd just come out of the confessional booth in a church. A weight had lifted from my shoulders. Just talking to another human being and admitting the truth had been such a relief. I remember thinking how hard it must be for doctors, knowing all of these intimate things about people – some of whom they inevitably know personally – and having to keep it all to themselves.

Self-harming, then, had been a symptom of depression. Depression is a deeply personal experience, however widely it seems to strike. In my case, the important thing to emphasise is that I hadn't known I was depressed. It had happened to me, it was acting on me, but I was so hyper-focused on my own distress that I couldn't see it for what it was. I blamed myself for the way I felt. And perhaps that is depression's true power. Its ability to seep in unnoticed and slowly steal your air.

I went back to Brum and started taking my pills. The ones for my blood pressure started working straight away. I felt a little less agitated overall but the effect was minimal. The only real difference was in my hands and feet. They got colder a lot quicker. The antidepressants, on the other hand, took a long time to do anything at all. The label said I had to wait two-to-four weeks before the effects would begin but the more days that passed without any tangible change in my mood, the less and less I had any faith in these tiny white pills.

But I do remember exactly when they kicked in. About three weeks later I was standing in a long queue, waiting to register for an Archaeology class. Without warning I started feeling sick. I looked around for the nearest loo. Where could I quickly run off to if I suddenly had to vomit? There was nothing in either direction but long empty corridors. The feeling grew and grew but stopped just short of making me physically sick. It swept up and down my body, a wave of nausea building up its own rhythm. My mouth watered and my throat clenched up. But the sensation would always ebb away right before it peaked. I had never felt like that before, it was like riding a roller coaster while standing still. By the time I'd reached the front of the queue, it had gone away completely.

After that the SSRIs started to make themselves known. I began daydreaming much more than I used to. I'd be sitting at my desk studying when my mind would inexplicably wander to something else. I'd sit back in my chair and stare at the wall for a bit, then push my books away and put some music on. I'd look at myself in the mirror and notice that my pupils were dilated. Big wide black holes where little pinpricks used to be. They were permanently open, not adjusting to the light around them anymore — just letting in as much light as possible. On other occasions, I'd be reading a book or looking out of the window and for no reason at all I'd start smiling. I didn't know what I was smiling about. There was no particular happy thought in my head. But there was a happy buzz inside me, somewhere, humming out from an unknown source. Day by day, this happened more and more. The smiles came automatically, in the same way you can't help but laugh when someone tickles you. I had the sensation of being able to just let go and enjoy the ride.

So far, so good — right?

A few months passed. And that sense of being tickled took on a new aspect. At night, when I was lying awake in bed, I would sometimes feel like I'd been submerged in a warm pool of joy. But it wasn't happiness as I'd ever known it before. It came from its own place and it felt alien. There were times when I would feel a tingling sensation at the front of my brain, just under my forehead. Like I was being tickled by an insect with dozens of prickly legs crawling around in my skull. Unsettling but exhilarating at the same time, it fixed my face in a permanent grin. I would stare up at the ceiling as I floated motionless in ...what? Mental ecstasy? As I floated there, everything about it felt wrong. The muscles in my face were being lifted by a third party. The smile was quite literally being raised. And not by me. It wasn't my happiness. I was just responding to stimulus. And the stimulus came and went without rhyme or reason.

During the day, the daydreaming got so powerful that I felt like a sleepwalker. I always knew the Seroxat was doing its thing when my pupils went as wide as saucers. From that point onwards, my mind moved further and further away from the present moment. I would find, sometimes, that I'd been sitting in a chair for a couple of hours − thinking nothing, doing nothing − completely unaware of the time that had passed, but filled with absolute contentment. I wasn't bothered about anything or anyone. I wasn't even aware of myself.

All of this came in waves. Pockets of concentrated happiness arrived at intervals throughout the day. And because these highs were steadily getting higher, the lows were feeling all the lower by comparison. When the SSRIs receded, the loneliness came flooding back in, colder and more bitter than before.

The culmination of all this emotional up-and-down was a night in my bedroom just a few weeks before my final exams. University had been a long, tough march and the last six months had started to feel like a road that led to nowhere. It was past midnight. I was sat cross-legged on the carpet, very drunk, holding a kitchen knife in one hand and a telephone in the other. To convince myself I meant business, I took a few more pills than I should have done – double the dosage for the blood pressure, double the amount of Seroxat – and called up my best friend, miles and miles away at another university. When he answered the phone, I told him I was holding a butcher's knife. And could he give me just one good reason why I shouldn't kill myself right now?

What a terrible position to put him in. What a mountain of selfishness I had climbed. I cringe to recall this moment. But it's important to share it with you because his answer was transformative. My friend thought for a moment, then said quite simply: 'because I'd miss you'.

Four basic words. Simple words. Maybe even obvious words. But these are four words that men can go an entire lifetime without ever saying to each other. Emotional silence, repression, deflection – call it whatever you want – is a very real problem between men. Who knows how many times a kind word from one man to another could have made all the difference in life? Who knows how many times that word is never, ever spoken. And a life gets lost? What I do know is that in my country, the United Kingdom, suicide is the biggest killer of men under the age of 45. That is a harrowing statistic – an epidemic. And I know it all stems from this basic inability to speak openly and honestly when it counts.

For me, those four words made the difference. My friend convinced me to put away the knife, stop drinking and go to bed. So that's what I did. And a few days later, he came all the way up to Birmingham to spend the next week with me. It felt like a real turning point. I decided to stop taking the Seroxat and the blood-pressure pills. I dug in hard for my final week of revision. Two weeks of exams passed by in one intense blur and before I knew it, university was over. There was one final week of loafing around ahead of me, before everyone left the Edgbaston campus for good.

I'd like to end this chapter here but there's one final episode I have to mention. You're supposed to come off antidepressants gradually. I ignored this and stopped taking them all at once. The result, for me, was one last relapse in that final week of university. Everyone else was in party mode and celebrations were kicking off on all sides. There was a Graduation Ball on campus that everyone was going to, including the small group of classmates and housemates I'd come to know over the last three years. But I didn't feel like celebrating with any of them. I was on a real come-down. They all went out to the big event in their tuxedos and ball gowns while I stayed at home, prostrate on the sofa. I remember watching *A Touch Of Evil*, lying there in the flickering blue light of the TV screen, slowly working my way through a crate of Boddingtons. I was looking forward to leaving this place. And these people. Let them all have their pointless party with their fake friends and their empty conversations. I was finally done with it all and I knew I wasn't missing a thing.

The truth is, of course, I was missing a defining moment of my youth. Graduating from uni is a rite of passage and one I'd never get back. There are photos from that night that my friends would later put into albums, mount inside frames and hang up on their walls. My face is missing from all of them. If only I could go back to that night, shake that young man off the sofa and convince him how important that fleeting, carefree time really was.

After coming off the antidepressants, I never took them again. And little by little my mental health improved on its own. Taking SSRIs had been an unpleasant experience for me but on some unknowable level, I believe they altered my brain chemistry. They did just enough to change my outlook for the better. The effects of that shift have been more or less permanent. I have never again sunk to such a low place. And depression of that magnitude has never visited me again.

# 15. Absinthe before breakfast

After graduation, I moved back to London. Back to my parents' house and into my old bedroom, with zero idea what I wanted to do next. I had a Bachelor's degree in Archaeology and English. On the archaeological side, I'd been on several excavations in the UK already to see where they would take me. On those digs I spent eight hours digging all day long with shovels and mattocks. Very often, we found nothing for weeks. The work felt a lot like manual labour and the British weather was routinely terrible. Could I do this for the rest of my life? I loved the ancient world but I quickly decided a life spent outdoors, digging and scraping around in the mud wasn't for me.

That left me with my English degree. I loved reading and writing. How could I get a job that would let me write for a living? I started applying for positions. Anything I could find that was related to writing. Editor. Subeditor. Journalist. Stenographer. I even remember applying to be a voiceover artist. Telling myself that to function in the real world I'd need to get a job that kept me away from people, I also applied to be a security guard in a local car park.

I got no response from any of these applications. Days turned into weeks. And then months. After two months of unemployment, I went down to the Jobseeker's Centre and signed on to the dole. I remember sitting upstairs in my room trying to make the most of all my free time. I read *Moby Dick*. And *Seven Pillars of Wisdom*. And all the while, my dad was getting more and more irate that his university-educated son was sitting at home on the dole reading books.

Around the same time, I had my first real relationship with the opposite sex. I still had a few friends up in Birmingham and I'd been going back up there every once in a while to hang out with them or go to their house parties. At one of these parties I met a girl called F who was in her fourth and final year of study. I stayed the night with her a few times and things moved quickly from there. I started going up to see her every other weekend, taking the National Express from the Victoria Bus Station.

This was a new and terrifying experience. Every time I'd seen F so far, it had been in the context of drinking. At a party, in the pub, at a barbecue. I'd always been a bit drunk in her presence and it made me feel calmer, more confident. And now that we were seeing each other more often I wanted to impress her at all costs. I was fearful that she'd see the real me – nervous, awkward, sweaty and blotchy – and suddenly find me weird and unattractive. The only way to stop that happening and keep up the act was to keep up the drinking. From the get-go, my bad rituals kicked back into gear. I felt it was the only way I could make the relationship last.

I have clear memories of the mornings before I caught the coach up north. I would get up around 5am. Shower, pack a bag, creep downstairs through the dark and silent house with an empty plastic Coke bottle in my hand. My dad kept a drinks cabinet in his dining room, which was strange, because he never drank anything from it. The alcohol was ostensibly there for guests, but they never touched it either. So it was always fully stocked. Johnny Walker. Bacardi. Gordon's. St-Remy. I had my pick of spirits. My dad never checked any of it so I felt comfortable syphoning off the supply, rotating between different bottles. There were always more bottles of Hennessy, for some reason, and I stole most often from those. I'd get a small funnel from my mum's cooking cupboard and fill my plastic bottle 90% full with the dark brown cognac. Then I'd add a splash of orange squash to fill it up to the top. The result was a secret supply of almost-neat alcohol.

Then began the road trip to Birmingham. On a good day it took about two hours, racing along on the motorway. And the trick was to take measured sips from the bottle the entire way up there, trying to make sure I was slowly reaching the perfect point of drunkenness by the time I arrived in the dingy hull of Digbeth bus station. F would be waiting for me out in the exit hall. Before I went through to meet her, I would rush into the men's toilets with my overnight bag and quickly brush my teeth at a sink. So that when I walked through the waiting room and we kissed, she wouldn't smell two hour's worth of carefully-consumed Hennessy on my breath.

This tactic worked. I would be happily drunk at that point and expertly hiding it. I would suggest we go to the pub. Or I'd produce a bottle of champagne from my bag and announce we were going home to drink it. Anything to keep me at the level I needed to be at so I wouldn't be my awkward, embarrassed self. I made this trip dozens of times and for that whole period, the relationship remained a long-distance thing.

Later, when F finished her fourth year and moved back to London, things with her would become more serious. I remember the first time I met her parents. I was petrified. Visiting them sober was out of the question. So I made sure I was at the perfect point of drunkenness as I sat down in their lounge. It was all a case of intricate timing and by that stage, I was well-practised at this. I made pleasant conversation as the four of us drank cups of tea and ate plates of cake. I even cracked a few jokes. I distinctly remember the sun shining in through the windows, specks of dust highlighted in yellow sunbeams, as the alcohol slowly started to wear off – wondering if I could make it through to the end of the experience without my mask falling off. In the end, I made it to the finish line undetected. I left the house having made a good impression and F never said anything that suggested she'd known I was sloshed. Neither did her mum or her dad. I'd learnt where the sweet spot was and how to hit it at the right moment.

About five months into unemployment, as I was almost convinced my degree had been a waste of time, I got a reply to a job ad asking me to come in for an interview. The role was at a well-known home shopping TV channel. They needed copywriters to write product descriptions on their website. It paid peanuts but I was thrilled to finally be in the running for a job, a real job doing something I actually wanted to do. I arranged the interview.

But one big question remained: how the hell was I going to go through with it? The very thought made me wither up inside. I pictured myself twitching and sweating in a chair, my face going redder and redder as my interviewers sat waiting for answers that were never coming. I thought about it all day and all night, lying awake in bed imagining all the different ways the interview would end in disaster.

When the day arrived, I gave in to this fear wholeheartedly and did the very worst thing. I got up in the morning, skipped breakfast, drank a bottle of red wine, got on a train and went straight into the interview. And to be honest, I don't remember much from that point. I know I went in there behaving like the opposite of my normal self. Calm, talkative, open, assured. I remember answers coming out of my mouth naturally. No hesitations. No sweating. No blushing.

A few days later, I got a phone call telling me I'd got the job. On one level, this was great news. I was finally employed. Doing something I knew I'd enjoy. But on another level I didn't recognise at the time, it was bad news. Because people (apparently) couldn't tell when I'd been drinking. I became convinced it was a deception I could comfortably control and it encouraged me to knock back more.

In my new job, everyone sat in an open-plan office. Desks were arranged into 'pods' for 4-5 people, all facing the centre to encourage collaboration. The company was fond of team-building activities. I remember two in particular. The first was a 'studio induction day', during which we had to go in front of the camera to see what it was like to be a TV presenter. The second was a two-day workshop focused on the company's very American values. Unsurprisingly, this was done in a very American way. At the end of it, a large circle was formed and each participant had to step into the centre of the circle to be 'appreciated' by the colleagues standing all around them. It was a social phobic's nightmare and I spent both events in a state of nervous paralysis, always waiting for my turn to step into the spotlight and hating every drawn-out second of exposure once I got there.

I started experimenting with natural calming remedies I'd found at the pharmacist. Surely something gentler than alcohol could calm me down? Sometimes on their own, sometimes together, I was taking white pills, pink pills, purple droplets you dissolved in water, yellow liquids you sprayed on your tongue. They contained extracts from plants like chamomile, dandelion, lavender, valerian, lemon balm, passionflower. I was also trying large daily doses of St John's Wort, the age-old herb for depression.

None of these made the slightest difference. They were all coated in hard sugary shells to make them easier to swallow. When you took them by the fistful, it was like gobbling down too many sweets. All they really did was fill me up with a sickly sweet sensation.

After one of those team-building days, I remember standing in a bar with a colleague. We were friendly at work and enjoyed a bit of banter. He said something like: 'I hate these things. They feel so fake and forced.' I agreed. But I'd also had enough drinks by then for drunken sincerity. I said something like: 'I've been taking pills all day long. I'm a nervous wreck. I can't stand being in a room with so many people, not knowing what's going to happen next. It's like torture for me. I've got some kind of phobia and I just can't take it.' Even as I said the words, I regretted them. The guy paused for a minute and looked at me funny, trying to decide if I was being serious or not. Then he said 'mate, I'm sorry, I had no idea'. We both moved the conversation on fairly quickly. And after that, in the cold hard light of day, I wished I'd said nothing at all. Because he was different after that and we never spoke to each other in the same breezy way again. We started avoiding each other in the hallways. There was a mutual air of awkwardness.

Over the next year or so I became slowly fearful of a very specific event. Whenever someone on my team went on holiday, they would come back to the office to something of a hero's welcome. People would bring over their cups of tea and their breakfasts and crowd around that person's desk, wanting to know where they went, what they saw, who they met, what they ate. It was a lovely social moment that brought the team closer together. But I grew to hate it, because I knew it would happen to me when I next came back from holiday. People would gather round me, expecting funny stories and interesting details. It was more social exposure than I was used to, condensed into 20 minutes. They'd sit around me, pouring their attention on top of me. And I knew I was going to drown in it.

So the cycle of anticipation kicked in again. Before I even went on holiday, I'd be thinking about my colleagues descending upon me when I returned. The future moment magnified itself, grew outside of itself. How could I come back and get through that moment without having a public meltdown? The answer was always booze.

But I needed the right kind of booze this time. Something powerful that would act quick and hard, to carry me through that crucial first half hour at work. I decided it had to be absinthe.

I'd moved out of home by then, into a basement in Stockwell badly converted into a one-bedroom flat. The place was overrun with damp. Slugs left sticky trails across the kitchen floor. It was in this basement, after coming home from a trip to see a friend in New York, that I opened up a bright green bottle of absinthe at 7am. I drank slugs of it from a shot glass, feeling the bitter herbs burning down my throat. Absinthe is about 80-90% strong and, on top of no breakfast, it didn't take long for the after-burners to start blazing. I remember walking to work, totally drunk, in the early morning drizzle, hoping this time that the effects would calm down a bit by the time I got through the front door.

When I arrived, as expected, people wanted to hear all about my trip. They congregated around my desk and asked me 100 different questions. I don't recall any of the answers I gave but I was more talkative, more composed, more casual than normal. I enjoyed being the centre of attention. But it was all short-lived. By 10 or 11am I was on a real downer, all bleary-eyed and sleepy at my desk with the rest of the workday to get through.

Drinking spilled over everywhere. I was drunk at my sister's wedding, before the ceremony even began. I had been chosen to be an usher and my entire family from the US and UK was coming together. I was overwhelmed by all the aunts and uncles and nephews and nieces, all the conversations and the happy act I was going to have to put on throughout the day. So I decided to start drinking champagne at 9am, making sure I was nice and drunk when the time came to speak to guests and guide them into their seats. Way before anyone else and well before midday, I was three sheets to the wind. There's a photo in my parents' house of me posing with my sister as she holds up her bouquet. My smiling face completely belies the truth. Mentally, I was gone. Somewhere else entirely. I was living a lie.

Some days, I developed a phobia of coming into work altogether. On those days, I needed a drink first thing in the morning or I wouldn't make it into the office at all. This wasn't a physical addiction. I didn't slip into DTs if I didn't get a drink. It was more of an emotional addiction. I needed the Dutch courage. Emotionally, when I was getting drunk at ungodly hours of the morning, I started finding the experience strangely thrilling too. Drinking at such a time is the last thing you're meant to do. It felt illicit and reckless: two words I'd rarely use to describe myself. It was a secret I perversely enjoyed keeping.

I once read somewhere that vodka is 'the alcoholic's choice' because it's easily disguised as water and has no odour. So I started drinking vodka as my spirit of choice. One day, I drank over half a bottle before I came into work. And let me just confirm it for you here: vodka is not odourless and no easier to conceal than any other spirit. I found this out the hard way, because people around me could suddenly smell the alcohol coming off me. 'Jesus, were you out last night? You reek of booze!' was the immediate response I got. That was all it took to plant a new seed in people's minds. *Hang on a minute, that's weird. Is Russell drinking too much? Is he drinking... in the morning?* Or at least, that's what I imagined them thinking. I started thinking too that now they would look for proof. If my reactions were ever so slightly slower. If my eyes were ever so slightly unfocused. I felt like I'd been caught out. I felt a sense of shame, like I'd been singled out as a deviant.

So I stopped drinking before work. Instead, I developed what was arguably an even more damaging strategy. I noticed one day when I'd had terrible insomnia the night before, that I was much less anxious. Lack of sleep seemed to make me care less about what was going on around me. It dulled the edges and brought my nerves down a level. So I started staying up late to deprive myself of sleep.

But the knock-on consequences were very serious. I become a zombie at work. I couldn't wait to get through the day and crawl into bed at night but I forced myself to stay up later and later and keep on doing it. I read books. I watched late-night TV. My work had stopped being challenging. I could write product descriptions for fake diamonds and hair products in my sleep by then. So although it made me dead on my feet during the day, I could still bash out my work with no real noticeable difference. And being sleep-deprived made me less prone to blushing. So I just kept on doing it.

One night, I stayed up until 6am, watching the sun slowly creep round the corners of my curtains. I didn't go to sleep at all that night and when I was standing in the shower, feeling dead inside my bones, with a sinking feeling that I had a whole day at work to face on zero hours of sleep, I started shaking all over. And then I was violently sick down the swirling plughole. I was amazed that lack of sleep could provoke such a visceral reaction.

One day at my desk I received a phone call from the HR Department. A lady on the other end asked me if I was free to meet up sometime soon as a matter of urgency. Because some of my team members had raised concerns about my drinking habits. They thought I drank too much too often and there was always a telltale odour of booze in my corner of the room. She sounded deadly frank and serious, as though this was an intervention and I was being given the opportunity to come along quietly, without a public struggle. My mind raced as I panicked and scrabbled to somehow defend myself. Blood rushed up into my face and turned me a familiar patchwork of crimson. Then I saw a group of my colleagues giggling behind their computers at the other end of the room. The HR lady's tone suddenly changed. *I'm only joking. Sorry, but the rest of your team put me up to it. No hard feelings, yeah?*

There were no hard feelings. What the rest of my team may not have appreciated was that they were, in fact, exactly right. I was developing a dangerous relationship with alcohol. I drank too much and slept too little for a good four years during my time at that home shopping channel. Towards the end of those four years, I broke up with my girlfriend. She felt a disconnect between us, something broken somewhere that couldn't be mended. In my final year there before I left, I met my future wife. And started making plans to move on to another job.

# 16. 'Live better! No sweat!'

It's a freezing morning in the middle of February. I'm sitting outside on a long brick wall, watching an endless stream of traffic fly past on Hammersmith Road. I'm 30 minutes early for an appointment, but instead of going into the office building behind me and waiting inside the warm lobby, I'm staying outdoors in the cold for as long as I can. I'm letting my fingers and toes go numb, feeling my nose tingling and my eyes watering. I'm out here because I want my body to cool down as much as possible before I enter the front reception and announce my arrival for an interview. Because the colder I am, the longer it will take for my body temperature to rise and the less likely I'll be to overheat and blush my way out of a potential new job. It won't make it unlikely, just a little less likely for maybe the first five or 10 minutes. It might be enough to make a good first impression before my blood fires up again and turns my face cherry-red. Half an hour of discomfort out here is worth the five minutes of grace I might gain in there. I'm just hoping one of the interviewers doesn't walk past right now and see me lurking out here like a weirdo.

Despite going in there half-frozen, I managed to hold myself together until the interview was over and I was offered the job two weeks later. I took it without question. The company was a huge internet provider, serving millions of people around the world. I felt like I'd taken a big step up. Now I was an Online Editor, responsible for writing digital features and promos. At that time, in 2005, the company and its website had become a household name. I couldn't wait to get started and begin afresh in a new office, with new people and new work and maybe a new-found confidence.

But almost straight away I realised the job I'd interviewed for and the job I was doing were two different things. I'd been told lots of writing needed to be done. Webpages had to be crafted, emails had to be composed. But for the first few months I saw precious little of that. Things didn't really need to be written so much as sold. The company had lots of commercial partners, most of them high-street retailers. As it turned out, my job was to reach out to those retailers and ask them what their latest deals were. Then get those deals posted on our website. This meant no real writing at all. But an awful lot of talking instead. On the phone. While everyone around me listened in.

All. Day. Long.

I'd somehow jumped out of the frying pan and into the fire. I didn't like talking on the phone at the best of times, always finding it hard to make conversations flow. Especially in a professional setting, when every word you said counted so much. Whenever I had to do any admin over the phone — speak to my bank, for example — I'd fallen into the habit of writing out what I wanted to say on a piece of paper, so I could have it there in front of me and at least fake a sense of fluency. But here at work, everyone could see me at my desk. I couldn't read my lines off a pre-written script. No one else was doing that. In fact, no one else seemed to find this hard. They were all naturals on the phone. A personable phone manner meant everything, here. And I was absolutely awful at it.

How could I have walked blindly into this? Had the role been missold to me? Had I not paid complete attention to the details, being too keen to take the first offer that came along? Either way, I now had to do something every day that made me feel sick inside.

When I punched in the number of a contact, I tried to forget all the people sitting within earshot of me. And it was just about impossible. Everyone could hear exactly what I was saying: even if they weren't looking my way or seeming to pay attention, as far as I was concerned, their attention was still on me. I could feel dozens of eyes flanking me on all sides, dozens of thoughts and judgements filling up the air around my head. A partner would pick up on the other end of the line, I would begin my stilted conversation and hear my own voice reverberating in my head as I fumbled my words and left awkward pauses. The whole office would fall eerily quiet as I heard nothing else but the words leaving my mouth in an uncontrolled stream, sounding louder than normal like I was shouting them across the floor, all the while acutely aware of myself and of other people's awareness of me.

The inevitable pattern formed. This was an experience that made me feel bad. I began to fear it. It became something I had to avoid. I started looking for ways to get around the phone calls. Maybe I could just email the partners? Or wait for them to call me? I would sit at my desk, knowing I had to make these calls but would be physically unable to make my hand pick up the receiver. Every part of me was mired in inertia as thoughts looped round my mind. **You should call now.** *But I can't.* **You should call now.** *But I can't.* **You should call now.** *But I can't.* Monday morning would roll around and I would do this for hours, telling myself I'd definitely make a few calls after lunch. Then I told myself I'd get it done by the end of the day. And that became getting it done by Wednesday. OK, so I would absolutely do it by Friday. Alright, too late now, it would have to be without a shadow of a doubt on the following Monday. This went on for a while and my work began to suffer. My team noticed I wasn't pulling my weight.

And then there were the times when the partners would actually come in for a visit. I'd have to meet them in person and shake their hands. When I get nervous, my hands quickly grow wet with sweat. The more I think about it, the wetter they get, until visible droplets of moisture are beading on my fingertips. When someone first meets me and reaches out to shake my hand, I'm the guy who wipes his palm against his trousers before clasping yours in a half-hearted, half-regretful kind of way. And why the regret? Because I know, when you feel my warm sweat touch your dry skin, a part of you will recoil. Either physically (I once shook hands with a woman who pulled her hand out of mine with a shock) or mentally (I once shook hands with a man who narrowed his eyes to look me up and down with distaste). I regret that I'm putting you in this position, but what can I do? A handshake, in the corporate world, is unavoidable. It's like saying 'please' and 'thank you' or 'bless you' after a sneeze. It's socially expected. People make quick judgements from a handshake. Too soft, you come across passive. Too hard, you come across aggressive. Wet and faltering, you just come across — odd. A handshake became something I only gave under duress. I never reached out my hand first. I tried to skirt around the moment as often as possible. Which, I suppose, made me seem detached and unfriendly.

It got to the point where I grew tired of this. Tired of my own body. Tired of the same old dread that came in the lead-up to a handshake. Tired of the judgement, imagined or otherwise, it provoked in others.

So I went to the pharmacist and scoured the shelves for anything that would help with excessive sweating. I found a treatment called Driclor. It was packaged up just like an antiperspirant but it claimed to do much more than your average supermarket roll-on. Most antiperspirants contain small amounts of aluminium chloride but Driclor contains much more. When you put this chemical compound on top of your skin, it reacts with your sweat and forms a gel. This gel blocks up your pores and prevents more sweat from coming out. I tried it on my underarms a few times first and it seemed to work pretty well. So I started rolling it across the palms of my hands and up and down my fingers, too, before I went to bed at night. And I have to say: for the next few weeks my hands were pleasantly dry. I went to work, shook hands freely, felt genuinely more confident with partners and clients at close quarters.

So far so good. But aluminium chloride is an irritant. If it comes into contact with water it turns into hydrochloric acid. That's why you have to put it on at night, so it gets 8 hours or so to seep into your pores and completely dry before you wash off any remaining traces of it in the morning. Your skin will never be fully dry. Even when you're not visibly sweating, there is still moisture inside your skin. Hence there's always some form of irritation with Driclor. At least, there always was with me. It started with itching that got so intense it kept me awake at night. I would scratch at my armpits, drag my nails across the tingling palms of my hands. This, of course, made the itching worse. Eventually, my scratching broke the skin and the chemicals started to burn even deeper. My armpits felt like they'd been scalded by hot water. My hands got red and swollen. So I stopped using the Driclor until my skin healed up. Then I'd use it again until the burns came back. Then I'd stop. Then I'd start. Yet another cycle to inhabit.

If something seems too good to be true, it's usually just that. There is no miracle cure, only a delay of symptoms. That's what alcohol did. And it's what Driclor was doing now. So after a while I threw it in the bin. It had always been a temporary answer. Not the answer.

When checking the Driclor website recently, I was surprised how openly it calls out the social effects of excess sweating (or *hyperhydrosis*, as they call it). They talk about 'the quality of life' of the people 'affected by this syndrome' – how 'it can cause emotional stress, making more difficult the normal development of activities on the occupational, personal and social stage, producing the creation of a vicious circle.' When's the last time you heard that kind of language used to sell an antiperspirant? Quality of life? Emotional stress? Vicious circles? It doesn't just acknowledge the psychology behind the symptom but the personal fallout from it, too. It makes this condition more acceptable. Something sufferers can live with. The Driclor slogan, in fact, is this: 'Live better! No sweat!'

You might argue Driclor is just exploiting the fears of its customers. But the plain speaking cuts to the heart of the issue. It's encouraging. And I wish there was some similarly honest language out there about blushing. I'm still looking for it.

It certainly wasn't there 15 years ago. I remember searching online in desperation for some kind of solace or guidance on blushing. I couldn't find anything apart from a single book written by an NHS doctor. I ordered it and eagerly waited for it to arrive in the post. I was certain it would contain some insight or advice that would change my life for the better. It turned out to be a short and disappointing read, written by someone far removed from the problems he was discussing. First, clinically, the author explained the biology behind blushing. Then he showed the emotional impact of blushing, using testimonials from anonymous blushers that — at the very least — made me feel a little less alone in the world. But when he suggested coping methods for blushing, everything simplified down to a level suitable for children. Advice like this:

*When you feel anxious, stop and take a long deep breath. You'll be amazed how a deep breath will calm and relax your body. Make sure you drink lots of water throughout the day, to stay hydrated and keep your body temperature stable. Wear more make-up in the situations that make you blush the most. Knowing the blush is less visible will make you feel more confident.*

I couldn't believe what I was reading. How mistaken this GP was on the everyday realities of blushing. For me, at least, breathing deeply has never helped me calm down, in any situation. I know people advocate breathing routines for generalised anxiety but for social anxiety, there's rarely any time to put this structured breathing into action before an anxious situation begins. Drinking water is good for you but it doesn't dim my blush response. I can drink litres of water all day long and still blush for England. As for wearing make-up; this just seemed to reaffirm that blushing was somehow a female problem that could be solved with a simple dab of cover-up.

But you know what? I was so desperate at the time that I still tried it. I went out and bought some concealer to put on my face to see if it would hide all the redness. It changed the colour of my skin, for sure, but it made me look like a badly painted waxwork doll. It was obvious I'd smeared make-up all over my face, just like it was obvious when I'd been drinking early morning shots of 'undetectable' vodka. I couldn't go out of the house looking like that. People would notice and comment on it more than the blushing itself. As I looked in the mirror at my crudely painted face, I could feel it getting hotter and hotter by the minute.

So my sweaty hands stayed sweaty. And my red skin continued to blush. Everyone in my new office noticed my nerves and found me aloof, a misfit, a loner – or that's the internal narrative I had in my head. When people went out for lunch together, I would go and hide in the toilets until they'd left the building so I wouldn't have to sit with them through a blush-filled hour. I was avoiding phone calls, avoiding partners, avoiding colleagues.

My manager, a woman in her early forties, started taking notice of my meek behaviour. She was everything I was not: confident, loud, gregarious, with a supreme belief in herself and her talent. This was her default state and if she came across anyone else who wasn't like her, it simply did not compute. I was so noticeably unlike her that she took a special interest in me. During our weekly direct reports, she would sit back in her chair and regard me with curiosity. Like a funny little specimen she didn't know quite what to do with. Who was this young man who still blushed like a little boy? Who shuffled in his seat and couldn't look her in the eye for more than a few seconds at a time? When her curiosity peaked, it turned into a kind of cruelty.

One day she told me breezily that I needed to up my game. And the way to do it was to start speaking at our morning announcements. These happened every Monday, when the whole company came together and a representative from each team took the floor to give an update. 'I've decided it's going to be you speaking for our department over the next few weeks. Because it will be good for you.' She paused, thought and gave a little smile. 'And because I know you'll hate it.'

I tried not to react. I suppose she saw herself as a motivator, a mentor pushing me outside my comfort zone. She had a beneficent look on her face, as though her tough love would do me some real good and one day I'd thank her for it. From my end, though, she looked exactly like a cat who'd caught a mouse, and was having fun playing with it.

I left the room and the black zeppelin slowly appeared on the horizon. There it was, looming just a few days away, the moment when I would have to stand up and address 50-odd people in the middle of a crowded office floor. It was an immovable threat, casting a long shadow over me. And there was no way to get around it.

I dealt with that challenge the only way I knew how. I stewed about it all day and all night for a week and when the day finally came round for me to make myself heard in the Monday morning announcements, I made sure I stayed up all night and only went to bed around dawn. I slept fitfully for one hour, then got up and blearily made my way into work. I was delirious and felt like I was moving underwater, crawling slowly through treacle. But the desired mental effect had been reached. I'd slipped into a hazy state of calm that only comes to me with complete exhaustion.

When everybody filled up the room and my cue came to get up and give my five-minute speech, I did it with measured confidence. In truth, I was on autopilot and practically sleepwalking. I'd been rehearsing every word I wanted to say for days and I knew the whole thing by rote. But I remember a sea of faces looking back at me with quiet surprise, watching me speak up in a way I'd never done before. It was as though they were seeing a new person for the first time.

It felt good. And the massive sense of relief when it was over felt even better. But I'd paid a high price. Very soon, the elation would wear off and I'd have a full day of work to get through on just a single hour of sleep. I'd be watching the clock tick forwards all day long, counting down the minutes and the hours. Avoiding people and phone calls because any form of conversation now just gave me a pounding headache. By 5pm I'd be utterly ruined and then, next Monday morning, I'd have to go through the entire charade all over again.

Later that same day, my boss sent me an email. She meant it to be genuine, I think. She must have felt she was doing the right thing. It ran something like this: *I want to say a big well done for giving everyone your update this morning. I'm so glad you're starting to find your way into your role and from here, you can only go from strength to strength. Everyone was so surprised you spoke so well. And you didn't even go red once! Bravo!*

When I read that message, the only thing that felt genuine was a massive lack of empathy. I felt like I was being spoken to like a 10-year-old. My boss had no idea who I really was, what was really going on inside of me, what lengths I'd gone to just to be able to stand up in front of our colleagues like this. Five minutes of public speaking apparently made all the difference? Now I was going from strength to strength and not a shrinking, struggling wallflower? Did she think I was being bashful on purpose, that I could in fact be perfectly calm if I really wanted to? If I only tried a bit harder? Was this whole awkward thing just a stubborn phase, a rut I'd fallen into? If I really just put my mind to it and simply stopped blushing, could I too be a successful leader just like her one day?

A nerve had been touched and I was overreacting to a degree. But I remember being furious at her message. She'd taken an intrinsic part of who I was — one I wrestled with daily, one that troubled me deeply — and trivialised it to almost nothing. She didn't understand. Nobody understood. How could they?

I didn't reply to her email. Full of frustration, I deleted it. And the next day, after a long night of restorative sleep, I started looking for my next job.

# 17. The biting point

It took me a few months to land one. I fired off applications and didn't hear anything back for weeks at a time. So in the interim, to give me something else to focus on, I decided it was probably time to learn how to drive.

It's perfectly possible to live in London without ever owning a car. Londoners are super-reliant on buses and trains and when those don't work we jump on bicycles or walk. I was 26 by now and I'd never been behind the wheel of a car, partly because I couldn't afford to buy one but mostly because I didn't need one. It was more a case of wanting a driver's licence, an important piece of ID, and giving myself a new challenge to work towards.

I signed up for lessons with the AA. My instructor was a little Spanish man with a thick black moustache called Antonio. After an initial lesson down a sidestreet all about switching gears and clutch control, we went straight out onto the main roads with thousands of other drivers in central London traffic. Antonio's approach was to throw you in at the deep end. I was taking my lessons right after work, usually in the dark as streams of cars made their way in and out of the city. He would lead us directly into the very worst spots: London Bridge, Parliament Square, King's Road, Kensington High Street. So much sensory input pouring in from all sides; my eyes darting between pedestrians, vehicles, road signs, traffic lights; my ears straining out for horns, sirens, pelican crossings; my feet feeling tentatively for every last vibration in the pedals at my feet. Cars racing towards me, double deckers pulling out in front of me, motorbikes whizzing past me before I could even see them approaching in my mirrors. Everybody driving so impatiently and aggressively and every move I made among them had to be perfectly timed and inch-perfect. An hour of this usually sent my senses into overdrive. And then into a kind of shut-down. I would slip into tunnel vision, a thousand-yard stare, so absorbed in what I was doing I often didn't hear Antonio telling me where to go next.

In short, for someone as tightly wired as me, driving was a perfect storm. It wasn't what I'd expected at all. Why, in these precision 21st century machines, were there so many ways to make a mistake? Stop with your foot off the clutch while in gear, the engine stalls. Miss the biting point – a position you can only find by feeling for vibrations coming through the clutch – and the car won't move. Miss the biting point on a hill and you're in a whole new world of trouble. I can't remember the number of times I found myself balanced on a steep London hilltop, revving the engine hard and slowly releasing the clutch, only to roll backwards a few inches, again and again, getting closer and closer to the bonnet of the outraged driver trapped on the slope behind me.

I know I'm not alone here. Hill starts in manual cars are a rite of passage for anyone learning to drive. But I found everything else that came with driving a bit of an ordeal, too. Knowing when to pull out into a constant flow of traffic. Having the spatial awareness to weave in and out of parked cars without scraping against them. Parallel parking while other drivers sat still and watched my every move, chomping at the bit to get past me. I came to these lessons straight from the office, already strung out from long days in an environment I'd grown to hate. To then get into a car and have London attack me from all sides – it all felt a bit much. By the time each lesson ended, I was shaking all over and my body was soaked in sweat.

And so driving, too, became something I was afraid of. And I started to avoid it. I'd paid for a batch of lessons upfront and the rules were, if you couldn't make a particular lesson you lost the money you'd paid for it. But that didn't deter me. On a bad day, when the time came for a driving lesson, I'd call Antonio and make up a story — I had to stay late at work, or all my trains had been cancelled — so I could skip the session and go home. I didn't do it all the time. But I started doing it more and more. Enough for Antonio to grow suspicious.

One day when we were waiting on a hill to enter a busy road of traffic, I had my foot poised on the clutch, one hand clamped on the steering wheel, one hand gripping the handbrake. And my whole leg started shaking. It went into a spasm, my foot slipped off the pedal, I stalled spectacularly a couple of times before we juddered out uncertainly into the traffic. Antonio looked out of his window for a minute, thinking. He usually tried to ignore my nerves and focus on the encouragement. But this time he came out with it straight. *It's good to be cautious but you are too cautious and it affects your body.* He looked at me and waggled his black moustache. *There is a vitamin you can take. Your GP will know it. It stops the shaking. It makes you more comfortable. I think, to pass your test, you will need one of these little vitamins.*

What he called a vitamin, my GP called a beta blocker. I went to the doctor, described my troubles with driving and asked for anything that might reduce the trembling in my muscles. He prescribed a box of Propranolol. And that was the first time I ever took it. One pill before every lesson gave an instant improvement. My heart stopped racing, my body stopped shaking, I concentrated less on my nerves and more on the task of controlling the car. I made sounder judgements. I was able to think ahead. It made all the difference and fast-tracked me towards my driving test.

And when the time to take the test came, I took two pills before going out on the roads for good measure. I took the test close to my mum and dad's house in Sutton. Antonio and I had decided that taking the test in suburban streets, after so many hours negotiating the hectic traffic of central London, would make everything much easier. And he was right. Now I understood why he'd forced me down congested roads night after night. Sutton was almost tranquil by comparison or maybe the beta blockers had just made me feel that way. Whatever the truth, I passed the test first time with just two minor faults. I was amazed and I think Antonio was too.

But the thing was, now I had a driver's licence and no car. And I wouldn't buy a car until I became a parent almost eight years later. Getting out on the road in the weeks and months after you first pass your test is crucial. It's when you consolidate your skills and build up your confidence behind the wheel. When I did finally get back in the driver's seat, I felt like a learner driver all over again. I was rusty and tense, full of pent-up panic. Beta blockers wouldn't help me now. How could I possibly take one every time I needed to go and drive somewhere? A fear of driving slowly crept back. Racing along a dual carriageway, I kept thinking how the slightest stupid mistake on my part could send me into a head-on smash with dozens of other vehicles. Especially when I was on the motorway and especially once I'd become a father. Speeding forwards at 70mph, I'd have visions of horrific pile-ups flashing before my eyes. Graphic accidents would fight for my attention and I'd find it harder and harder to concentrate on the road. I'd sit there squeezing the steering wheel hard, wondering how the hell I'd ever reach my destination without causing some kind of awful mass collision that would make people shudder that night when they saw the 10 o'clock news.

At first, I looked for ways to avoid driving again. I'd take the train or the bus or ask my wife to drive instead. But gradually, the more I got out there and simply drove from A to B, out of a new-found necessity as a dad, the weaker the fear became. These days, the panic I used to feel has lost its edge. It's still there, quickening my pulse sometimes and stiffening my back, but it's grown duller by the year. Repetition and routine have worn it down to a point where I can just about handle it. But to tell you the truth – if you gave me the choice, I'd still rather not drive. I just don't enjoy doing it. It puts me into an uncomfortably heightened state, trapped somewhere between fight and flight, and I'd rather avoid that stress.

But going back to 2006: I'd moved out of my basement flat now, I'd been sharing a few flats with a few different people I knew. I got a phone call one day from a recruiter asking about my background. My interests. And if perhaps I liked playing video games? He was looking for a copywriter to fill a role at a gaming company. A really well-known global gaming company. I'd be writing the instruction manuals that came with video games, he told me. Did that interest me at all? And did I want to come in sometime for an interview?

I'd been a gamer all through my teens and I jumped at the chance (while my heart jumped into my throat at the thought of another interview). I still had a few beta blockers left over from my driving lessons. The temptation to take one before the interview was just too great. I wanted a change of scene so badly, so I downed a pill an hour before the interview and went into it feeling steady. I remember an hour-long chat running over into two hours while I talked and talked and was perfectly amiable and said all the right things. The beta blockers really did work wonders, sometimes. Just a few days later I was offered the job.

Would I have got that role if I hadn't taken that pill? Who can say. But my gut instinct is no, I wouldn't have got past the interview, I would have blushed, seized up, made the wrong impression, pushed myself off the shortlist. Looking back at moments like that I find I can almost justify a strategic reliance on meds. I wasn't taking them all the time, only in the situations that really mattered. If they helped me through some of the key moments of my life, then so be it. They weren't harming me or anyone else. And nobody needed to know about it.

Then I remind myself how thoughts like that sit at the top of a slippery slope. Taking a pill once in a while quickly slides into once a week, once a day, just for important presentations, just for important conversations, just for any conversation. Physical addiction is one thing. But this is emotional addiction and it is, I think, even more powerful.

The good news, though, was I now worked with a team of writers and designers. For the most part they were quiet, more introverted types. They preferred a calmer working space. They liked to keep the overhead lights turned down low and I found the hushed gloom soothing. I've always felt more comfortable in low-level light and here was a place where my co-workers seemed to feel the same. I was at home here. The work was more creative and I brought a new creativity to it.

But when I had to go into the wider Marketing department, down a stairwell and into the adjoining building, it became a different story. They had a bigger, louder, much brighter environment over there. Lots of conversations and a faster pace. When you entered the room through its double doors, it was like stumbling out onto a floodlit stage. People turned around to see who'd come in. Once inside I'd always keep my eyes on my goal: someone's desk I was heading to at the other end of the floor, maybe, or a meeting room off to the side. I'd quickly thread my way through the tables and sofas, trying to reach my destination without making eye contact or calling any attention to myself. And then it would happen, someone would stop me dead in my tracks to ask me a question or strike up some chat. The trigger would pull with an interior ping and my blush would erupt. If it wasn't my day, the person who stopped me would comment on it. That I could more or less handle by now. But if it wasn't my week, they'd decide to bring some more people along for the ride. *Hey: Rob, Rich, Rita! Look how red Russell's gone!*

And so I often found myself in the same position you found me in at the start of this book. A man afraid to enter a room, pacing around outside in the hallway with one eye fixed on a shut door he can't bring himself to open. A new kind of snare was closing around me. I'd always showed physical avoidance but this was threatening to become a physical inability, a new kind of constraint I hadn't seen coming. I'd managed to find freedom in this new job but at the same time I'd managed to lose it, too.

It made me ask myself that bigger question again: how can I change all of this for good? Not make it better, more tolerable, but get rid of the discomfort forever? The only answer I could see was a medical one. I started hunting around online again for anything relevant and I soon discovered a specialist medical procedure called an Endoscopic Thoracic Sympathectomy (ETS). In the simplest terms, it's an operation that stops the body's blush response and drastically reduces sweating. Both reactions are closely tied to and controlled by a nerve running through your chest. If you go inside the body and cut that nerve in two, it's like you've removed the conductor between two electrical circuits. The signals that cause blushing, sweating, trembling and a wildly thumping heart — they still fire off as normal, but they can't be received and translated into all the physical symptoms of panic. With these symptoms silenced, there's no reason to fear them any more or avoid the situations and people that used to cause them. The vicious circle, for the first time ever, would be magically broken. And a whole new kind of life would be allowed to flood in and wash it away for good. I've said before there are no miracle cures, but this one sounded close.

I researched some more and saw the operation was available on the NHS. But to qualify for it, you had to prove to a consultant that the physical effects of anxiety were significantly lowering the quality of your life. Being permanently unemployed, being clinically depressed, being an active suicide risk — these were the debilitating criteria they were looking for. I didn't truly meet any of these, so my chances of a funded operation seemed pretty slim. That didn't stop me brooding over it, though, and dreaming about the life-changing results it could bring. Maybe I could pay for it myself somehow? I started looking into the costs.

That led me to reading all about the risks. To reach the correct nerve, hidden deep inside your chest, surgeons have to cut open your armpit and collapse one of your lungs. They enter your ribcage with endoscopic scissors and when they find the right spot, a few millimetres away from your spine, they sever the offending nerve, exit the body and sew up your wound. Then they do the same thing through the armpit on the other side of your body. All the while, you're completely unconscious under general anaesthetic.

For a lot of people the outcome seemed good. They reported less blushing, less sweating, more confidence, more participation in everyday life. But I also read about a lot of things going wrong. Too many things going wrong. Some people suffered brain damage during surgery. A few people died. Others had unexpected and long-lasting nerve damage affecting other parts of their bodies, from drooping eyelids and frozen facial muscles, to numbness and paralysis in arms, hands, legs and feet. But the most common problem by far was something called 'compensatory sweating'. When you cut the nerve that makes you sweat and blush, your nervous system apparently tries to reroute itself. Patients who were initially happy with their newly dry skin soon reported uncontrollable sweating in places they'd never sweated before. All over their backs, across their stomachs, up and down their legs, liberally covering their faces. There were people who described an ecstatic absence of blushing, who soon developed something called 'harlequin syndrome' — flushing of the skin on one side of the face. It's so symmetrical that it looks like a line has been drawn down the middle of your forehead, nose and chin: one side bright red, the other side not. ETS was supposed to cure a problem but in many cases it just created a bigger one. The internet was full of people expressing their regret, warning others to think twice before they signed up for this unpredictable and irreversible procedure.

So I abandoned the idea. It was a last resort and way too risky. Ruling it out left me deflated. But maybe there was some wisdom here, in the complexity of the human body and the many ways we misunderstand it. Remove part of a nerve to kill something undesirable and who knows how many desirable things you might kill along with it? My situation often felt intolerable. Yet here I was, tolerating it. My nerves made me miserable but if I thought about it hard enough and rationally enough, weren't there times when they were doing me some kind of favour? Giving me more self-awareness? More empathy? Showing me more meaning in the small things that might otherwise be missed? This was the genetic hand I'd been dealt and if I tried to deal myself a different one on the operating table, there was a very real chance I'd damage more than just my body. And come to know what intolerable really did mean, as a result.

That's what I was telling myself on good days. On bad days, I was instinctively looking for escape routes. If it wasn't going to be surgery, could it still be medication? Who cared if chemicals were a short fix for a long-term problem. I needed something to relieve the pressure in the here-and-now and something better than a simple doctor's prescription.

Lots of people go through a druggy phase and writing about it feels passé. But there is an important link between fragile mental health and substance abuse. And why some people feel the need to turn, almost inexorably, towards illegal drugs. My experience had been an on-off experiment all through my twenties. I already knew the many benefits of alcohol. Maybe, if I found the right drug, it could work for me in the same way?

I'd always hated weed. It just made me feel dopey and sick, apart from one night in the USA when I smoked some homegrown stuff with friends that washed my world in vivid colours and filled me with a physical joy I haven't felt before or since. All other times, it just turned me into a puking zombie. Ecstasy was always fun on the dance floor, with music thumping and lights flashing all around. It lifted me out of myself and immersed me in mental bliss. But as soon as I stumbled out of a club into the pale dawn light, there was a price to be paid. A week's worth of serotonin had all been used up in one go, making the next few days hollow and bleak as my brain tried to refill its supply. I took too much ketamine once and I spent a few hours inside the dreaded K Hole, trapped in my own body like a prisoner looking out at the rest of the world from the wrong side of a TV. Cocaine gave me the instant confidence I always lacked and, for a while, became the biggest draw. It absorbed all my fear and burned it up as fuel. While it lasted, coke solved just about all my problems. But all my problems weren't confined to Friday and Saturday nights. And, of course, it's a drug that notoriously bites back. All through the daytime, for days after I took it, my nerves would be dialled up to 11. I'd be twitchy and paranoid while my system tried to reset itself and find its way back to some kind of balance.

The only drug that never came at an obvious personal price for me was psilocybin, or magic mushrooms. When I ate them and they made the sky turn purple or the wallpaper come alive or turned the faces of my friends into gleaming multicoloured gemstones, my brain wasn't being slowed down, sped up, drowned out or even frozen – it was being rebooted, somehow. After a trip on mushrooms I would always slip into a night of deep, peaceful, regenerative sleep. When I woke up the next morning I would feel mentally refreshed, cleaned-up from the inside out, as though someone had sorted through the sprawling mess of my memory banks and filed everything back into careful order overnight.

But what was I going to do, walk around for the rest of my life high on mushrooms? If anything, what I learnt from drugs was how little I really knew about myself. Behind my consciousness were things that weren't me. They could be brought to the fore or pushed into the background with chemicals but did I really have any control over any of them at all? My unconscious mind did as it pleased. So why did mine decide that I must blush, that I must sweat, that I must tremble? Why did it autonomously bring all of these ingredients together, to make me fear the presence of people? I was looking for answers. But they weren't going to come from drugs that gave my subconscious self even more free rein.

My job was going well. Despite regular moments of social anxiety, I liked my colleagues. My boss accepted me for who I was, with no attempts to train my awkwardness out of me. I found my work fulfilling. So fulfilling, in fact, that I stayed in the role for the next six years. Long enough to move in with my girlfriend, and ask her to marry me. These were happy times and looking back on the years that took me from my twenties into my thirties, I realise how important they were for me. Slowly, in increments and almost without realising, I was getting more comfortable in my skin, getting closer to a new point somewhere nearer the centre. And one memory in particular seems to confirm this for me.

One year, we had our company Christmas party in a pub. The

place had been booked for the night and some entertainment was arranged, including a live comedian who liked to move around the room and pick on people in the audience. He got laughs by singling you out, poking fun at you, pulling you up on stage to make you act out some kind of silly task. I got dragged into it but was drunk enough by that time not to care anymore. My anxiety was sufficiently masked to let me spend a few minutes out in the spotlight. Later, when the show was over, I remember going downstairs to the bar and seeing another writer on my team coming into the pub through the front doors. He was a softly spoken guy. Very clever, very good with words. I'd seen him blush before in meetings and felt a natural kind of kinship with him. He joined me at the bar.

'Is it all over?' he asked.

I wasn't totally sure what he meant. 'Is what all over?'

'The comedy gig.'

'Oh, yeah. It ended half an hour ago.'

'Good,' he replied. And ordered himself another pint.

I got curious.

'Weren't you here?' I asked. He grimaced and shook his head.

'God no. I popped into the pub over the road. Had a drink on my own. I can't stand that kind of stuff.'

He said it like it was perfectly normal. Like any reasonable person would find that situation disagreeable and leave the building, alone, to hide out across the street until it was all over and done with. I remember pausing, taking stock, looking at the two of us in the glowing mirror behind the barman. For the first time in a long time I felt like maybe I wasn't so unusual after all.

# 18. Wedding nerves

Towards the end of my stint in video games, as I turned 30, my girlfriend and I bought a flat together. We moved out to the edge of south London, into the leafy suburbs of Kingston. Life felt much calmer there, compared to the rush of urban Clapham. When you walked around, you could hear the birds chirping and tweeting in the trees.

During our first summer in the flat, we took a week's holiday to New York. We were coming through passport control at La Guardia, where some new security measures had just been put in place. All five fingerprints on your right hand had to be scanned and recorded on a digital touchscreen before you could enter the USA. Like many people I get apprehensive when I pass through airport security, feeling like I've done something wrong or I'm hiding a secret.

But I get much more worked up. By the time it was my turn to be fingerprinted, my heart rate was up and my hands had started to sweat. A severe-looking man behind a checkpoint desk ordered me to put my index finger onto the glass screen. I did it and watched the monitor blip a few times, trying to pick up a reading.

'Take it off,' he barked at me.

I took it off.

'Put it back on.'

I put my finger back on top of the glass and held it there. And the system failed, again, to scan my skin through the layer of moisture coating my fingertip. The man looked me up and down with growing impatience.

'Do your next finger! Put it on the screen!'

I pressed my middle finger onto the screen and nothing was registered. As I lifted my hand away, I saw beads of sweat sitting on the surface of the glass, so I wiped it off with the cuff of my jumper. It left a wet smear. The man opposite me was becoming livid, with fury surging in his eyes. His computer said no. I was screwing up his day.

'I can't get a reading! It's not working!'

He looked at the smear, slowly evaporating off the glass.

'Why are your hands so wet?'

I shrugged and looked back at the hundreds of people snaking behind me, waiting to get on with their lives. I blushed deeply, feeling singled out, full of a childish sense of shame. The man watched me as I put my fingers out, one at a time, on top of the glass touchpad again. No response at all. Just more moisture glistening on top of the screen.

'What's wrong with you?' he hissed.

I kid you not, this man was that rude. I wanted to shout back in his face, ask him what gave him the right to speak to total strangers like that. But I was too embarrassed. And I'd been through US customs many times before. The best thing to do was keep quiet and let the officials do their thing. This official glared at me with detest and loudly sucked his teeth, then punched at some buttons on his keyboard.

'Just go through. Get through!' he shouted through his booth, motioning me past like a bad smell. We went through the gates and continued on our trip. But I spent the rest of the week worrying about what would happen on my way back through La Guardia to get home. They wouldn't try to take my fingerprints again, would they? Not on the way out. But what if they did? What if the exact same thing happened again? The feeling stuck with me beyond that, too. For a few years to come, it made me think twice about going to the US. If there was a chance I'd be publicly humiliated every time we touched down in an airport, that was a chance I'd rather not take.

In New York, we'd planned a week of sightseeing. All the classic touristy stuff. Times Square. The Statue of Liberty. The Bronx Zoo. The Empire State Building. But secretly, I'd also been planning something else. At the top of the Empire State I was going to ask my girlfriend to marry me.

Popping the question would be nerve-racking enough but getting to the top of the skyscraper was even more so. To get to the roof you have to take a series of lifts between 102 floors. And each lift has its own queue, meaning you queue up for 20 minutes, go up a few floors, queue for another 20 minutes (and so on). My girlfriend didn't know what was coming and was getting more and more fed up with our slow ascent to the top. In truth, she'd been indifferent to this part of the trip. I was the one who'd made her come here. I was the one who'd sold it in as a sight not be missed. We spent a good hour slowly moving up the building with my nerves stretching tighter and tighter with every passing minute. It soon felt like a special form of agony: just standing there – knowing, waiting, sweating.

When we finally reached the square viewing platform on the rooftop, it was very hot. In the middle of a heatwave, close to 100°F. The viewing platform was much smaller than I'd expected and crammed to bursting point. You could walk around all four sides in 60 seconds flat if people hadn't been standing everywhere, pressed up against the barriers and filling every available space as they tried to get a look at the city far below. The roof was uncovered and the sun was beating down hard. We shuffled slowly around the platform, taking photos here and there through all the bodies. I was looking for a gap in the crowd, some quiet corner where I could pull my girlfriend aside and do the deed. I told myself I'd do it on our first circuit of the platform. But we went around once and I chickened out. So I persuaded her to go back around a second time. And then a third time. All the while, I was having runaway thoughts of abandoning the whole idea and just getting us out of this place. Do it somewhere else. Do it in a bar, a restaurant, somewhere you'll be more relaxed. But this feeling was all too familiar. It was the same feeling that made me cancel my driving lessons, that made me walk past closed doors instead of opening them. It was welling up inside me, predictable as ever. And this time I told myself to stuff it back down as far as it would possibly go. I committed to the moment, grabbed my girlfriend's hand and we both stopped still in the middle of everyone.

'Ugh, get off me! Why is your hand so wet?'

(I thought of the guy in passport control, shouting at me across his desk.) She didn't mean it, she was hot and fed up, I managed to pull her further aside and quietly asked her to marry me and she was incredulous, at first. I had to ask a few more times before the message sank in. Then she smiled. And nodded quietly.

And before I knew it we were back in London, the weeks and months were flying past and we were knee-deep in wedding plans. Visiting venues and caterers, tasting wedding cakes, choosing flowers, writing invites, trying on suits and dresses. The biting point had become the tipping point. Things were shifting. I was creeping into my thirties, becoming an adult. And the change felt good.

Although I already knew by then the wedding day itself would be a challenge. We'd both be the centre of attention all day long. All those photos and videos, all the family and friends, the hundreds of hands I'd have to shake, the speech I'd have to give. The black zeppelin floated up and took its place in my mind. I started fearing everything well in advance, but it frustrated me even more deeply this time. My wedding was supposed to be one of the best days of my life. It shouldn't be something to dread. I felt split in half. Rationally, I was excited and looking forward to it all. Irrationally, I was terrified of losing control and letting myself down, my fiancée down, everyone I knew down. The contradiction grew as the wedding drew closer.

The night before we got married, my fiancée slept in a hotel and I spent the night on my own at home. My nerves jangled and I couldn't sleep. At dawn, I got up and went for a long run to clear my mind and lower my blood pressure. Then, as arranged, my groomsmen slowly started to arrive at my flat and we slowly started to drink champagne. On the way to the venue, in the back of the cab, I took a few tablets of Propranolol. Once there, as guests arrived in a steady stream and I welcomed them into the ceremony room, my groomsmen were telling me things but I couldn't hear what they were saying. I forgot to go and have my prep interview with the registrars, so they had to come and get me and we rushed through it all in a back-room. Then the ceremony happened, in a slow-motion blur, with every muscle in my body locked tight. I remember the utter silence, how loud our voices sounded as we repeated our vows. After the ceremony and the official photos, the alcohol started flowing and I started to feel more comfortable. Beer first and then a lot more champagne before dinner. I was measuring and administering. I was in my parents' kitchen all over again, in the early morning light, carefully filling an old Coke bottle with just the right amount.

My speech was coming up soon, so when no-one was looking I took another dose of Propranolol. During dinner, I drank several glasses of wine. By the time I stood up to give the groom's speech, I'd hit the sweet spot. Drunk enough to tell some good jokes, calm enough to keep my train of thought and hold my paper notes without them trembling wildly in my hand. After the speech, we cut the cake, had our first dance. And then the zeppelin broke free of its tether and drifted away. The pressure eased and the weight disappeared. Now it was just a matter of drinking and dancing and having a good time.

Imagine a rubber band pulled back on your finger and stretched out taut, straining hard as you hold it in place. When you release it, the pent-up energy sends it flying away from you right across the room. That was me in the closing hours of my wedding. The nervous stress that had drawn out all day long stopped suddenly and I lost control of my balancing act. My friends were lining up the tumblers of whisky. The shots of cognac. And I drank them all as soon as they'd been poured. As the end of the night drew near the beta blockers, the booze and the sensory overload had consumed me. I was rocking back and forth on my heels, stupendously drunk. As people gave me their heartfelt goodbyes and left to go home, I could barely stand up. I had to be helped out of the venue, into the back of a cab, up the stairs of my hotel to the bridal suite. Where I was violently sick down the toilet. Twice.

My wife knows what I'm like and how nervous I get. She knows the struggle and the symptoms and why I sometimes do the things that I do. But she wasn't happy that night, to say the very least. I'd pushed it too hard. In the morning, after a few hours of broken sleep, with the absolute hangover from hell, she questioned me on the last few hours of the night before in meticulous detail. To prove to her I could remember it all.

Which, it turned out, I could. Twenty-four hours later all was (mostly) forgiven and when we both look back on our wedding night now, we're able to laugh. But she was absolutely right: why had I overdone things? Why did I have no true self control? I'd been elated all day long but also engaged in a private battle of self-preservation. In the end, the two had clashed — and exploded.

We honeymooned in the Seychelles. We'd booked ourselves into a little resort on an idyllic private island. Swaying palm trees against the tropical sun, giant tortoises roaming around on the beach. But on the day we arrived we were told in person by the resort manager that swimming in the ocean was strictly off-limits. Under no circumstances was anyone in the resort to leave the beach and enter the open water. Why? Because just the day before, on the neighbouring island a few miles away, a man had been killed by a shark. He was newly married, had just checked in on honeymoon with his wife – and got torn to pieces in front of her eyes by a Great White. The island we had chosen was totally remote. No mobile reception, no internet in any of the rooms. This local story got picked up by the international news networks, somehow. The headline on websites and newspapers ran like this:

## BRITISH MAN EATEN BY SHARK ON SEYCHELLES HONEYMOON

Because the victim hadn't been named, all my friends and family at home started sending us panicked texts and emails. And because we were completely unplugged in a rustic beach cabin, we didn't receive any of those messages until a couple of days later. At which point, my continued existence surprised everyone. But it was a sobering thought. As I laid in our cabin watching the blue waves roll past, I thought about the hidden killer swimming somewhere underneath. What if that had been me? What if life had suddenly ended, just like that, in the mouth of a passing shark?

Later, when we got back home, I decided my job wasn't challenging me. I'd reached a point where the work felt routine. I had itchy feet and a sense of regret I might hold later on if I got too comfortable in an office where everyone kept the noise hushed and the lights down low. I was and still am lucky to work in an industry that lends itself well to freelancing. There were many pens-for-hire who'd successfully struck out on their own. The idea had always appealed to me. I'd daydreamed about it one too many times at work already: about what it would be like to do things my own way, to charge my own rates, to throw away the safety net and see what happened next.

So I quit my job without any other work lined up. It felt risky and out of character but also like the right time to make an experiment. I had a modest mortgage and just enough savings. My wife and I shared a joint income. We had no children yet. I told everyone I knew I was going freelance. A few weeks passed while I stared out into the abyss with no referrals, no leads, nothing at all coming my way.

But then, just before my time was up, an old colleague recommended me to a charity she worked with. They needed a writer, fast. I had a phone interview and sent over a few samples of work. They booked me up there and then for my first gig.

# 19. Going solo

Freelancing brings a lot of freedom. It lets you choose who you work with and when you work with them. In some ways it makes you feel like the master of your own destiny. But it comes with a lot of restrictions, too. Sometimes you feel like you can't turn down work. Like you shouldn't take a holiday. Like your working hours don't end at the close of business on Friday. You have to look after your own taxes, your own pension, your own business insurance. You have to promote yourself. And biggest of all, for someone like me, it's best if you're a people person. You are now the face of your own business, responsible for winning work and building a reputation. Contractors live in a competitive market where first impressions really do count. People pay good money for their services, recommending them to friends and colleagues if they do a good job. Once they get a new contract they can't sit back. They have to be active, present and forthright in everything they do. When you're working permanently in a company, it's easier (perhaps) to slot into position and wait for things to come to you. As a contractor, your role is temporary. And because you are temporary and some people in the business don't know you they will often bypass you. To get your work done to the best possible level you have to let them know you're there so you can keep connecting the dots. AKA a go-getter. AKA a people person.

My first job was with a homelessness charity, where I had to get to know a lot of new people quickly. I sat next to the departmental boss, which I found awkward at first. She could see my screen and she liked small talk. The offices were hot, cramped and unloved. The air-con never worked and there were more bodies than desks. The still, suffocating air in that building made me feel uncomfortable all the time, always on the edge of a blush. But I made a conscious effort to be sociable. I started conversations with everyone, instead of waiting for them to get to know me. I played badminton with some people after work. But I still had a strong aversion to eating meals with others. That was one worry I just couldn't get round. So every day I went out to get some quick lunch on my own, taking a long walk around the Brutalist buildings of Farringdon and the Barbican. All in all I worked at this charity for about five months, writing fundraising copy and trying my hardest to make new connections.

I befriended one guy, a young shaggy-haired planner who'd taken this job straight out of university. Let's call him Planner Guy. He was a bit of a musician, a pianist who was knowledgeable about classical music. I didn't know a great deal on that subject and enjoyed chatting to him about composers and instruments. It was all easy and we just seemed to click. On my last day in the office, when my contract was up, Planner Guy passed me in the corridor and I reminded him I'd be leaving later that day. 'Oh god, it's your last day already? No worries. I'll come down later and say a proper goodbye,' he said.

Simple words. But probably the last words I wish he'd said. I've always hated office goodbyes. When people come over to your desk and linger, a little group hovering around you, wanting you to say something memorable or give a little speech before you leave the place. He was going to come down on his own and say goodbye but what if he picked up a few other people along the way? Or what if, once he got to my desk, other people overheard his goodbye and drifted over in my direction, circling round my chair, all eyes on me, all expectations pointing squarely at me? It would be just like those moments when I came back from holiday to a gang of curious workmates. Those moments, not so long ago, I couldn't even be part of without getting drunk before I turned up at my desk in the morning. In all fairness to Planner Guy, all he'd done was tell me he'd come and find me to say farewell. In all fairness to my phobia, he'd just told it to go on high alert. And from that point onwards time started dragging like a block of stone. For the rest of the day I grew more and more tense. Waiting for him to turn up. Waiting for the predictable moment when I'd break out in a sweat and turn red and make an awful last impression on everyone.

So, at the end of the workday when I saw him enter the floor on the other side of the room – and stop for a minute to have a word with someone else – instinct took over, sending me out of my chair and straight into the toilets. I locked myself in a cubicle and sat down in silence. He would come up to my desk and it would look like I was in a meeting somewhere or just too busy to be at my seat. I'd arranged some leaving drinks for later that night, anyway, and knew I'd be more comfortable with all the goodbyes once I had a few drinks inside of me. I'd speak to him properly then.

I stayed in the cubicle for 30 minutes, I think, feeling like more and more of a loser all the time. When I finally slunk out and back into my chair, he was nowhere to be seen. Some of us did go out for drinks after work that night. But Planner Guy wasn't there. I wondered where he was, guessing he'd made other plans already, which is why he'd wanted to say goodbye in the office. The more I drank, the more I loosened up and the easier it got to talk to everyone – the worse I felt about snubbing a perfectly nice human being while sober. People remember you by the way you leave things, a voice kept telling me in the back of my head. After I left the charity offices I never saw or heard from Planner Guy again.

Something similar happened in my next role. I took a job writing for a big UK telecoms brand, based in a huge open-plan office full of hundreds of hotdesks. You had to sit in a different place every day, making it easier to disappear in a sea of faces. But there are always people who don't want to disappear at work. Or let anyone else do it. One young guy in my new team always wanted to go out for lunch. Not go out and get some lunch but go out and sit in a local restaurant and spend an hour or two eating a pricey meal, usually washed down with a few pints of beer. Let's call this man Developer Dude. Initially, I went out with Developer Dude and his small crew of colleagues almost every day. I was trying to make a good impression and fit in and every time we sat down at a table to eat, I went through my internal struggle like clockwork. Every minute feeling like an hour; taking fake trips to the loo just to kill some time; drinking just enough beer to make my skin feel hot and flushed for the rest of the day but not enough beer to put me at ease in their company. They truly didn't know how hard I found it to sit with them and go through this process every day. It was steadily exhausting me. I dreaded this shared lunch hour and tried to find a way to get out of it.

So I chose a familiar strategy: to be away from my desk when Developer Dude came over at lunchtime. I'd leave the office early to have lunch on my own. And for a little while, that worked. All I got from him was the odd comment later on in the day. Where were you at lunch? We had an awesome green curry. Couple of cheeky beers, too. Don't miss out tomorrow. I would tell him I'd been on a phone call or something or maybe I'd met up with an old friend for lunch. Then one morning he caught me early as I arrived at my desk. *Lunch today, mate? We're going to the pub. I know you love a pub lunch.* I really didn't love a pub lunch. And I really didn't want to go. But I didn't have an excuse prepared and as he stood there, grinning expectantly, I paused for a few seconds too long and missed my window for escape. So I just said *yeah sure* to get him off my back, hoping he'd forget or else the day would get busy later on and everyone's plans would change. But as 1pm drew near I saw him at the other end of the room getting his little group together. I did my usual disappearing trick; I got up, walked away, and hid in the toilets for half an hour. When I came back out, Developer Dude was long gone. But there was a note waiting for me on my desk. He'd scribbled this on a Post-It: 'Where are you? We've gone to the pub. Here's my number. Call me and I'll order for you.' I stood there blinking at it. So now I had to call him up and deliver some kind of half-arsed excuse in person, while all the others listened in as he tried to change my mind.

An internal monologue erupted inside of me. *Jesus Christ! Why am I being hounded like this? Why am I being forced to call this guy, a kid just out of school, someone I barely even know, to justify the way I want to spend my lunch hour? Why is it so important that I join you all for lunch? Do you have any self awareness whatsoever? Can you not see when someone is unkeen, when someone — shock horror — doesn't want to do what you want to do? Why am I always so polite and obliging, why can't I just come out with it and say no? Why can't people just leave me alone? I know I'm being antisocial but why does that give you the right to tell me where I have to go and eat my food? Who asked you to order my lunch for me? Who asked you to go out for lunch every single day like it's some kind of unmissable event? Don't you ever have anything better to do? Just let me do my own thing! Just give me one hour of the day to do my own thing in peace!*

In the end I rang him up and went through an interminable phone call. I rambled off an awkward excuse while he sounded like a disappointed parent. He'd kept a seat for me and everything, he said. I was going to miss out on some awesome craft beers, he said. I told him it was too late now and I wasn't going to come. It was toe-curling and absurd. But it didn't stop him asking me to go out for lunch every day after that, too. I couldn't decide anymore who was being unreasonable. Was this deliberate or just the way he was? (A question I imagine people asking themselves about me.)

The work at this telecoms company was fun and interesting. But after six months or so, I didn't renew my contract. A friend of a friend mentioned my name to a recruiter in a large British fashion house. I had a Skype interview with their Head of Copy and agreed to start there a week later.

At this luxury retailer I was thrown into a very different world that made Developer Dude seem trivial. In their meticulously designed offices, full of monochrome black and white, everything and everyone had to make an impact. Mode was paramount and character was everything. The people here were larger than life and egos were always clashing, throwing off sparks. But above all else, in this place, fashion was art. And art was here to change the world. It was the most socially intense environment. Intellectually challenging, too. On both fronts I had to be at my absolute best every day, always turned up to 11.

I started going for long 10km runs every morning before work — in the winter months, getting up well before sunrise — to burn up as much nervous energy as possible before the working day ahead. I was the freelancer in the room, the consultant, the expert, and the work was piled onto my plate. I suppose by now I was already feeling the first pangs of 'imposter syndrome'. The feeling that you're unqualified for the job at hand and only just managing to hide it. The language of high fashion very often flew straight over my head. I had to quietly Google all of the industry-speak. What if these people gave me something I really couldn't do? What if I got something totally wrong and damaged their brand? Most importantly, when social anxiety struck at an inescapable moment, what were they going to think of me? In this uber-slick environment where everyone walked around coolly, dressed like they were ready to step into a photoshoot? What would they think when I lost my grip in public and how much longer would they keep me around?

The Copy Department in that company was exclusively female. A team of 20 or so young women. I was the only man in the room and it made me feel uncomfortable. Once a month the department held a team meeting. An agenda was drawn up in advance and an email went around asking if you had anything to bring to the team's attention. If you did, you were invited to address the group when the meeting happened, as it always did, in the middle of the open-plan office. People usually pulled up chairs or perched on desks. If you were the one speaking up, all eyes were on you.

A few months in I added something to the agenda. Because on the outside I wanted to be seen as a contributor, as someone who was joining in. And on the inside I wanted to start seeing myself as someone who walked towards my fear. I habitually ran away from fear. It was time I at least tried to confront some of my behavioural tics, the same old signals that had traversed my brain a million times before and left a well-worn groove in their wake. That groove was too easy to follow. So I put my name and my update down on the list, to follow a harder path. The meeting was a whole week away and I tried to be optimistic. I told myself I felt fine about it and tried to push it from my mind even though it stayed, hovering, at the edges.

I was still ignoring it on the day of the meeting. The time came to go and gather around some desks. I joined the team, we all chatted for a minute or two, then our manager shushed everyone and kicked the meeting off.

As different people stepped forward to say their piece I started asking myself why I'd ever chosen to do this. The other speakers couldn't have looked more at home. They didn't fumble a single word, every thought was fully formed, if someone asked them a question they had a zippy, friendly response like they were talking to a neighbour over their garden fence. How could so many people be so good at this? Did they have some kind of confidence gene? How could they be so utterly immune to blushing? Was it physically impossible for them? How wonderful it would be if I was unable to blush. Think of the possibilities. Think of the person I could be.

As the meeting moved its focus from one person to the next, panic started filling my veins. The voices faded out, I wasn't hearing what anyone else said, I was just thinking about the moment, coming any minute now, when the group focus would fall on me. There was no way out of this now. People weren't looking at me yet but once they were, I knew exactly what would happen. How tiring it was, going through the same process for what felt like the ten-millionth time. I was powerless, tied down on familiar tracks, just waiting for the train to speed through and hit.

The meeting was handed over to me and through thick air I started talking to the room. I could feel the blotches arriving quickly on my face, spots of fire growing hotter and hotter. People's eyes started moving, I couldn't help but notice it, tracking down my face and across my neck. I started seeing confused glances, whether they were really there or not. I started hearing what I assumed everyone else would be thinking: *What's happening to you? What's wrong with your face?* By the time I'd finished rambling through my update, my face felt like an inferno. I was sweating through my shirt. This really had gone 100% wrong, my social anxiety had whiplashed with a vengeance and here I was, laid bare as a weird nervous wreck in front of all the people I'd been brought in to impress.

At the end of these meetings, it was customary to agree on who would host it next. The atmosphere had clogged up now and, perhaps to relieve some tension, the young woman who'd hosted this meeting said breezily: 'Oh, I think it should be Russell'. And everyone laughed. I laughed too. But inside, I was dying and desperate to get away from there, where people couldn't look at my twitching, red-splattered face. I agreed I would host the next meeting and everyone slowly dispersed. My plan was to disappear from sight and try to cool myself down. I could already feel the dip that comes after a sudden and pointless burst of adrenaline and that's when I most want to spend some time alone. To leave the room, I had to walk by the manager's desk. She called me over as I passed and I immediately thought: here we go, she's going to ask me if I'm OK, if I have some kind of social or physical problem that maybe she can help me with or give me some patronising advice like a mother speaking to her shy little boy.

But she didn't do any of that. She simply said:

'Thanks for volunteering today. You don't have to run the next meeting if you don't want to. I think the girls were being a bit out of order.'

I was thankful. And my knee-jerk reaction was to grab this waiver with both hands and never repeat that scenario again. But how long could I carry on doing this? Seriously: how long could I avoid every moment of social pressure, day in and day out? Now that everyone had seen me blush, now they knew I found it hard to speak in public, the toughest part was probably over. The edge had come off and now I could be more like my real self. The fact was, my real self blushed. That was never going to change. Maybe next time the experience would be slightly less traumatic. Even if it got 1% easier, wasn't that still something worth aiming for?

I told the boss I was happy to host the next meeting and a month later, that's what I did. But here's the thing: I don't remember anything about it. It can't have gone great but it can't have gone terribly, either. It's the terrible moments I remember and they stick with me for years. But I'm trying hard to remember this moment and I really can't. At all.

I take it as a positive sign. Social anxiety is essentially a lifetime of holding on to all the moments that other people throw away. Forgettable moments for them, unforgettable moments for you. But what's missing from that blank spot tells me more than any bad memory ever could. That was a point in the cycle where social anxiety had skipped a beat. Its mechanism had wobbled. All I needed were more and more of these forgotten moments, inconsequential moments that stayed inconsequential. If they started adding up, they could incrementally push the SAD out of its orbit, slowly pull it out of its groove.

At that time my wife fell pregnant with our first child. After a year in British fashion I gave notice on my contract. The plan was to take a couple of months off work, a rare luxury I could only enjoy as a freelancer. At no other time in my career have I stepped away from work for that long. It felt like a deep breath of fresh air. I imagined a world where things could always be that way, where you could just get on with life away from offices and people and blushing and stress. Fantasies, of course. Kind of like when you dream about winning the lottery. But we all need to fantasise every once in a while.

That was a strange, still time. The days were coasting past in the lead-up to our due date, feeling long and surreal. And they reached a new level of surreal when my son finally arrived, one week later, just a few days before Christmas.

# 20. Not about me

Right after my son was born, my wife was rushed into surgery to stop a dangerous haemorrhage. Someone put a wad of medical papers down in front of me. *Do you consent to these drugs, do you consent to this procedure?* In a daze I signed them all off as fast as I could. The doctor and midwife both disappeared and there I was, sitting alone, holding a baby boy in a bloodstained blanket. He'd stopped crying all of a sudden. I stared at him dumbfounded, frozen to my chair, while he stared back at me in total silence.

Most parents I know say the same thing. You're never truly ready to have children. There's no such thing as 'the right time'. But in the lead-up to birth, I'd been ready for months. We'd been through the NCT classes. We'd read the baby books. We'd bought the essentials. I felt as prepared as I'd ever be and, one week beyond our due date,

I was almost impatient to get on with it all. But now the big moment had finally arrived, in an empty delivery room right on the verge of Christmas, it hit me hard that I had absolutely no idea what I was doing. It was 10.30am, we'd been up all through the night, *Jingle Bell Rock* was jangling on a radio somewhere outside in the hallway, my wife was unconscious on an operating table and I was holding a gently shivering human being in my hands. How could I have possibly thought I was ready for any of this?

The feeling only got stronger when our son wouldn't breastfeed and wasn't putting on weight. We weren't allowed to leave the hospital for the next week. Even as things slowly improved, as my wife got back on her feet and my son learned how to feed, I had a gnawing fear of the moment when we'd finally bring him into our flat and the door would click shut behind us. That's when reality would truly dawn. There'd be no more nurses, no more professionals to help us through the delirium. The life of our helpless newborn baby would be squarely in our hands.

We went home on Christmas Day in the end, driving through deserted streets in streaming winter sunshine. My hands were wet on the steering wheel. It was the simplest of drives but I hadn't slept in close to 100 hours and my nerves were shredded. Just imagine having a crash now, I thought to myself, with a tiny baby sleeping in the back. What a stupid crash it would be. Into a concrete bollard or down the side of a parked car.

The first few months after that are still a blur for me. The baby slept with us in our room, waking every three hours to be fed. In between his feeds I remember the strange snuffling animal sounds he made all through the night. Grunting and growling, making it impossible for us to get to sleep – something we were both now desperate for. I'd always been one of those people who needs eight hours of rest every night. If I got anything less I'd be useless the next day. Washed out physically and mentally, struggling to get anything done. Now I was getting about four hours a night at best. And my wife was getting even less than that. But somehow she took it all in her stride. I don't know how she did it because in the beginning, the lack of sleep totally knocked me for six.

They say you build up a sleep debt for every hour of sleep you miss and those lost hours can only be repaid in kind: one hour taken out requires one hour put back in. If that's true, I ran up an enormous debt in the early months. And although the rate of loss slowed after a while, it never really stopped. I've been steadily losing sleep for years now, as parents do. The saving grace for me was that, somewhere along the line, my body clock reset itself. I got comfortable with five or six hours of sleep a night, something I once would have told you was impossible. Nowadays I've swung the other way. I can't sleep for eight hours anymore, even if I get the chance. My eyes ping open after six hours and that's it – my day has begun.

Why is any of this important? Because I think it reveals something important about the human body. When it's forced into new habits, it takes autonomous action and adapts. Parenthood is an adaptation. It's a slow act of metamorphosis and there's no doubt you come out on the other side of it a different person. Biochemically, you change, just as your child is continually changing. Every month brought something new from our son. The first smile. The first laugh. The first steps. The first words. Pretty soon, the first birthday. And then the first day at nursery. Through all of this I was growing alongside him.

I believe becoming a father helped me loosen the grip of social anxiety. Parenting puts you in a unique position, one that forces you to keep moving forwards. If my social anxiety had been one long act of avoidance, of irrational self-preservation, then parenting forced me to do the exact opposite. It was something that had to be met head-on, rationally, and it demanded genuine selflessness. It's this sense of self-sacrifice, I think, that makes or breaks you in the beginning. During my first year as a dad I often felt depersonalised, like all the things that defined me were slowly being erased. My spare time wasn't spare any more. My interests were no longer my interests. My priorities turned upside down. Which all sounds a bit obvious, now I'm writing it down. What exactly did I expect once a kid arrived on the scene? I suppose it's more proof I wasn't prepared for it, for the intensity of it, for the sheer non-stop nature of it. People don't give enough consideration to the first few months of parenting. It's a shock to the system with the power to break up relationships, end marriages, send people over the edge. Expecting parents can be perfectly happy until the baby arrives, then their entire world shifts with a force they hadn't reckoned for. For new mothers it can lead to postnatal depression, a very real and very dangerous thing. New dads get depressed about fatherhood, too, even if that feels like something that's easy to mock. Men have got it easy, so the narrative goes. They don't have to give birth, they don't have to breastfeed, their bodies won't be changed by childbirth. And all of this is true. But when life changes permanently it leaves deep marks, for men just as much as women. Having a child is a paradigm shift, one of those seismic moments in life that feels powerful enough to move the ground beneath your feet: a death in the family, a move to a new country, the beginning of a new career. To me, there was a time when this shift felt tectonic, like giant plates were giving way beneath me so the world could swallow me up. Simple things, like sitting down to read a book, weren't possible any more. Sleeping in late on weekends to catch up from a tough week? It had always been there, always taken for granted. And now it was gone for good.

This too shall pass. These are the truest of words. And all of these misgivings did eventually pass. But not with the passage of time. They only passed once I accepted I wasn't ready for them and I had to let my life change. Now I had a child to look after, it really wasn't about me anymore. I had less time and less energy for my own internal worries. My focus was completely redirected to the outside. And that for me was a potent thing.

I've never had Cognitive Behavioural Therapy (CBT), even though several doctors recommended it. It seemed at that point like I was getting my own special brand of CBT, anyway. Parenthood was forcing me down new neural pathways, marking out new routes, burning up my nervous energy in 100 different ways. While all this was happening I focused on my social anxiety less. It was still there, still bubbling away in the background. But I couldn't dwell on it like I used to. And dwelling is the oxygen that keeps social anxiety alive. By re-routing negative thought patterns, the vicious cycle was being disrupted again. Slipping further away from its core. Over the days, months and years that followed, I can genuinely say this made me a happier person.

By the time we had a daughter, three years later, I felt like my personality had been redesigned. As though I'd regained a clarity I'd been missing for years. Yes, it was twice as hard with another child. Yes, the demands doubled. But now it was twice the fun too. And a little girl is a very different thing to a little boy. Both kids gave us something unique every day, bringing all of our lives closer into balance. I'm a fairly pessimistic person and if you told me I'd be saying these things before I became a dad, I would have wrinkled up my nose and called it bullshit. All the more evidence that fatherhood fires off some kind of chemical reaction, I suppose, that alters who you are. Chemical change is the only thing strong enough to shift the way I feel, the way I think, the way I behave. More than a physical operation could, more than aluminium chloride on my skin could, more than taking beta blockers in secret or getting drunk in the morning ever could.

But at the same time, please don't get me wrong. There are some days when fatherhood brings out the worst in me. When I get up at 6am on a Sunday and it's pouring with rain outside and I have to find ways to keep my kids busy for six hours just to reach lunchtime – there are times when my mind drifts off to risky places. I start thinking how great it would be to have the house all to myself, to play my favourite music for hours, to buy the Sunday papers and spend the whole morning flicking my way through every page. At noon, why not just start drinking? There'd be nothing to stop me opening a bottle of whisky, clinking some ice into a tumbler, watching the amber Scotch fill the glass. I could walk around the house in my pyjamas, peeking out through the window blinds, hunt down some dusty storage boxes and look through all my old books. Later, I'd put a classic film on and see it from a whole new angle because I'm getting pretty drunk. Maybe then I'd get into a hot steaming bath.

And take my whisky with me. Isn't that what rock stars and artists do? Get sloshed in the bath? I'd spend all day doing things I never get to do anymore. All the things I shouldn't be doing. All the things I've left behind.

A self-indulgent, self-destructive tendency lurks within me. It's something addictive that doesn't care about consequences and I work hard to put it in check. I'm 40 years old now and it's the challenge, what isn't easy, that I'm looking for these days. Not what's easy, not the course of least resistance, not the path around or away from the obstacle. It's a feeling that's crept beyond fatherhood and, almost by stealth, changed the way I look at things.

Which means it's changed the way I look at social anxiety. They say that a change is as good as a rest. Becoming a dad is clearly one very big change and, speaking literally, the exact opposite of rest. But speaking figuratively, it's a change that's given me some new-found rest from social fear. I think about it less because I'm being forced to look in other directions. It gets less of my headspace, fewer opportunities to intrude into my thoughts. On top of that, I find my kids help me in social settings by naturally taking the limelight. They keep conversations moving, occasions rolling. After being with my children I find it easier somehow to spend time with adults. It doesn't hold the same level of terror for me anymore. Kids have thrown me into a network of other parents as well, people I already have a lot in common with. Children threw some rational weight against my irrational phobia and helped me push back against it. And slowly, the social anxiety that had mushroomed inside me for so long started getting squashed down around the edges.

But it isn't just this sense of diversion that helped me. It's also a sense of the future, of the potential. When I think back to when I was a twenty-something in a nightclub, punching a wall and trying to break my hand, or cutting my arms with a kitchen knife, or staying up into the small hours with a creeping desire to kill myself – I had no sense of tomorrow, of the things to come. Life was immediate, it was unfair and unfulfilling in the here and now. I felt that way because everything was defined by me and me alone. When life becomes bigger than you are, it gets redefined. You don't just find a new respect for the lives beyond yours, you find a new respect for your own. Little people depend on you now. You must keep yourself safe to keep them safe.

A couple of months after having our son, I went back to work. I was still a freelancer but something was niggling at me now, something was telling me I needed more permanence in my life. I'd need a bigger home soon, a bigger mortgage, a regular income. And I was tired of doing my own taxes. So I took a contract at an advertising agency. Luckily enough, it soon turned into a full-time position. Having spent most of my career working in-house or directly with clients, now it was time to see things from the agency side of the fence. I'd always wanted to work in advertising but it's hard to enter that world, unless you're coming from another agency. Freelancing had put my foot in the doorway. And now I was being invited to step inside. It felt like a career high.

# 21. New agency

Life in an agency can be exciting. When times are good – free lunches, free booze, international travel, global brands – it's close to exhilarating. Things move fast and sparkle as they go. When times aren't so good – late nights, weekend work, losing a pitch, losing a client – it's exhausting. Things slow right down and the sparkle fades. Everything inside an agency moves to the rhythm of this financial ebb and flow. Highs follow the lows. Lows follow the highs. Your employer's fortunes are always going up and down and the fluctuations are more or less constant.

The highs, when they come, can be truly high. Your work gets written about in the press. It wins awards. But the lows can be awful. Maybe your work bombs commercially, or people are made redundant. You'll find yourself at one extreme or the other, up high or down low, but seemingly never in between. Which means that sooner or later everything comes down to pressure and how you handle it. For some people this can produce the best work of their career. For others it can send their career off the rails.

I know what some of the low points were for me. I always struggled to find a balance between parenthood and my agency existence. Although work hours officially ended at 6pm, almost nobody went home then. There was always another email to send out, another piece of work that had to be ready first thing tomorrow. It meant I hardly ever saw my kids before bedtime. My wife bathed them, read them a book and by the time I got back from the other side of London they were fast asleep. At first I thought this was par for the course, that to get ahead and be a responsible dad you had to put in the hard work and the extra hours at the office. But then I thought about how quickly time passes, how it won't be long before my kids will bathe themselves and read their own books. And I realised that being a responsible dad was actually about being there for these moments, precisely because they won't last forever.

There were times when I had to take work home with me and do it on the weekend, instead of playing with my children. There were times when I had to stay up and work late into the night, losing more and more sleep. Or when I worked on four projects all at once, feeling smothered in stress and noticing tell-tale dips in my health. I'd start getting ulcers in my mouth. My throat would hurt when I swallowed. I got headaches at my desk as I stared at my flickering laptop, trying to ignore the notifications coming through on my phone. It was usually then, when I became acutely aware of the world moving faster than me, that I knew work was getting the better of me. There was a pattern to this and my wife could pinpoint when it happened. After two months without a break, I started to creak. The days got long and my reserves ran low. After eight weeks of running on a treadmill it felt like the agency was sucking up all of my life, so I had less and less of it to give to my family when I finally got home.

But this is hardly unique. Adland is rife with burnout. And alcoholism and drug abuse, for that matter. I've come across all of these in my career. But mostly it's the exhaustion that seems to penetrate everything. The sense that people are being worn down and chewed up. I worked with a young woman who quietly disappeared from the office one day. Simply there one minute and gone the next, signed off indefinitely because she'd had a nervous breakdown. I had a lot of empathy for her because she, too, was prone to blushing. English was her second language and I think it put her under some extra social pressure at times. She was very, very good at her job but one day something inside of her just broke. She was spirited away by the HR department and I never saw her again.

From time to time I hear the same thing about other people. So-and-so has been signed off work. Such-and-such has been sent home to recover. Sometimes you'll see the person again, sometimes you won't. And when you don't it usually can't be discussed by anyone for legal reasons.

I worked with one guy, a fellow freelancer at the time, who seemed to be sliding into alcoholism. He'd turn up at work looking red-eyed and hungover and you'd naturally assume he'd had a heavy one the night before. We've all had heavy nights and struggled through the next day at the office. But then you'd realise he was still wearing the same clothes he'd had on yesterday and it would dawn on you that he hadn't actually gone home that night. He hadn't even gone to sleep. He'd been drinking straight through until morning and came back into work. He was still drunk and would make it through the rest of the morning on strong coffee and banter. Then, at noon on the dot as the alcohol finally started to leave his system, he'd find some way to get back to the pub. And his own vicious cycle would start all over again.

I'd never seen anything like that up close before. There was drinking and then there was drinking and this kind of addiction put my own bad habits into the shade. But before we pass judgement, we have to remember that nothing is ever clear-cut. Addiction is always a symptom of something else. This man was under the same pressure as the rest of us. He had the same exhaustion slowly pulling him down. But he'd just had his second kid, too. He was in the eye of the storm back at home. His identity had shifted again and he seemed to be reeling from it. There were deeper problems going on beneath the surface – and again, I could empathise.

Because in theory, agency life should have been a recipe for disaster for me. In the very beginning I definitely drank more. A lot more. The first team I joined had an unofficial mantra: get all your work done by lunchtime, then go to the pub and don't come back. I was new to the culture and that was fine by me. It meant we didn't just have a few drinks and then go back to work, which always set my nerves on fire. We had a lot of drinks and stayed out instead, dousing my nerves completely. Pints and pints of beer followed by espresso martinis. If we did have to go back to the office, the drinking just continued. The project we were working on was top secret, it had a conflict of interest, meaning we were locked in a room on the ground floor and hidden away from the rest of the agency. We had cases of beer down there. Bottles of wine. Bottles of gin. We would get pissed all afternoon and I'd go home at 6pm feeling like it was 2am on a Friday night. I told myself I was just letting off steam in a stressful environment. This was advertising, this was just the way it was. I was easing myself into a new industry and a new team in a familiar way.

But this didn't last for long. After a while I realised I didn't like being half-cut in the office, trying to hide it from people. It was a short-term thrill but ultimately it just made things worse. So I stopped drinking in the daytime. I decided I wanted to make myself known at this agency, not hide away in a back room, hammered, doing just enough to get by. But I wasn't really sure how to do that because the more I got to know agency life outside of our secret little bunker room, the more intimidating I found it all. Expectations at this place were dialled up to their highest. You always had to be switched on. You had to bring your A-game to the table every day. Your work was under close scrutiny, creative goalposts were always moving, clients were coming into the office all the time and we were always preparing presentations for them.

In fact — later on, having escaped the hidden bunker and spent a year or two deeper in the agency — it felt like life had become one constant countdown to the next presentation. *The client's coming in tomorrow. Make sure the deck is ready.* For me, as you know, the worst feeling in the world is knowing that a moment of social performance is on its way; the zeppelin in my peripheral vision casts its long black shadow. But now there was a new kind of zeppelin to contend with, one that rose up out of the ground and hit you where you stood. Now there were moments when I had absolutely no notice at all. *Oh hey, can you just hop onto this call we're having in ten minutes and walk the client through all that stuff you did last month?* What could I possibly say to my colleagues at times like that? 'No' as I turned around and ran out of the building?

A lot of people make up an ad agency but I soon came to know one of the biggest things they all have in common. Designer, strategist, producer, writer: it doesn't matter who you are, it's not enough just to be good at what you do. It's the abilities that extend beyond your job description that keep your head above the water. A great deal of these come down to soft skills, your people skills. The most brilliant designer in the world won't make it very far if they can't communicate their ideas face-to-face. Inspiring writers aren't inspiring unless they can also inspire in person, in the flesh. Character and personality count for so much in this trade. They are the magic ingredients that create rapport, put clients at ease, push through the best work possible.

At first I hated this emphasis on talking, on schmoozing, on walking people through your ideas. It felt like the work was never allowed to speak for itself. You had to be the conduit, the mouthpiece, between the work and the customer. Explaining, persuading, selling. We live in a permanent state of elevator pitch. This is draining for introverts, let alone people with any degree of social anxiety. Add to this the busy open-plan office, the constant interruptions, the endless noise, the bright lights, the lack of anywhere quiet and still to go and sit down to contemplate your work — and it seems like advertising should have been a very special kind of hell.

But for me, it ended up feeling like a round of exposure therapy. I had no choice but to drop into the deep end and keep swimming. Every time I faced a new client or another presentation (I reasoned) a new neural path would open up. New roads would mark themselves out, old ones would close themselves off. Isn't that how a brain matures over months and years? The things we call experience and wisdom are really just a slow change of directions: water trickling one way across a rock, and as the shape of that rock gradually changes, the water diverting and trickling another way.

Every day became a challenge. But mostly in good ways. For the first time ever I had complete autonomy over my work. As long as it was ready for the client on time, I could do it however I wanted. From a desk, from a cafe, from my sofa at home. No one checked up on me unless they had to, there was no one breathing down my neck or micromanaging my every move (as I'd found in some of my other jobs). It was my responsibility to deliver the goods. Call it an honour system, of sorts, an unwritten agreement that time was yours to use as you saw fit, provided you came up with the quality. Not that we ever really had the luxury of time. Just about everything I was asked to do usually had to be done in half the time I'd done it in previous roles. Which sounds constraining but often it felt liberating.

And it forced me to do better work.

When my work was done I would go on client calls to talk through my writing. Or, to be precise, their writing designed for their brand. Before long I was leading some of these calls, gently steering the client. It's very unlike me to control a conversation, to take charge of it and push it in a certain direction. I've always been more of a listener. So this was uncomfortable. But by necessity I found myself doing it more. And by stealth, worrying about it less.

And then I started hitting more highs than lows. There were days when I felt like I was brimming with creative potential. Days when I was being given real opportunities to expand my horizons. When I was doing things that I would have thought were beyond me. I presented to the CEO of a global bank, on the top floor of a skyscraper in Hong Kong. I chaired a roundtable talk between top business leaders in Germany. I gave talks on copywriting to packed rooms of people (one of them about the potential of introverts). I became a manager. I became a mentor. I climbed the ladder from Senior, to Director, to Head of Copy and took on all the extras that came along with it: hiring, firing, politics, budgets.

Often I look back on this and ask myself how it was all possible. And I can't lie, those beta blockers did help. But the question still remains: how, with social anxiety, did I find my way there? Through a curious mix of time, immersion, a shifting personal landscape and a slow reaction to increasing pressure – it just sort of happened. On its own, slowly, like wind repositioning an entire desert dune, one grain of sand at a time. They say that people get a 'seven year itch' because that's how long it takes for every cell in the human body to replace itself. No one knows how many cells make up your body but the best guess is something close to 37 trillion. And they're always regrowing. So that every seven years, you literally become a new person. It's a principle that makes perfect sense to me, whether you notice it happening or not. Your mind, just like your body, travels through constant growth. One effect of growth is you shed parts of yourself along the way. I had grown more accustomed to pressure at home and at work, meaning the pressure of a social phobia – which, for such a long time, had felt so crippling – had dwindled.

But I wasn't in the clear and I doubted I ever would be. I still worried about social encounters, before they even happened. I still went bright red when someone talked to me, for no real reason at all, as they watched me blush and gave me a funny look, trying to figure out who'd done something wrong: me or them. I still berated myself about it for days afterwards. But now it just didn't happen as often.

With age I've gained perspective. I know that my kind of social anxiety doesn't stop me from living a fulfilling life. And I feel lucky for that. Because for a lot of people it's different. Their anxiety is more severe, their genetic code is less forgiving. For even more people still, mental illness makes everyday life and steady employment the biggest challenges they'll face. By comparison, I don't face the same challenges. I have a lot to be thankful for.

These days I'm more mindful of that than ever.

# 22. Social distance

Although agency life was an accelerator for me, professionally and personally, I only lasted in that environment for just over five years. Which seems to be the average for a lot of people. The pace and the pressure had done me good and pushed me into places I'd never been before. But it was all coming at a price. I'd never felt more tired, more wired, more distracted from life at home. I wanted to see my kids more. I wanted to get some decent sleep. I wanted my phone to stop buzzing and pinging at all hours of the day. I'd had a good run, met some great people and done some of my best work yet. But it was time to slow down and take stock. To just take a moment and remember to breathe.

I resigned from my role quite suddenly, without any of the next steps figured out. It was like a fuse going off. All of my energy abruptly stopped and I had nothing left to give. I didn't feel emotional when I walked into my manager's office and quit. It was calm, businesslike and over very quickly. But later on the same day, as I sat on some sofas typing out my formal resignation email, a senior woman I worked with came over and sat down next to me.

'How are you doing?' she asked.

'Oh I'm fine,' I answered, not looking up. I was distracted and not in the mood for small talk.

'Are you sure?' she continued. I stopped and looked up. 'Because it's like you're here with us right now. But you're not actually here at all.'

Wow. Words that shot straight to the bullseye. Did I really look that dejected? I thought I was just sat there typing an email. Did she know I'd already quit? I hadn't told anybody else yet. This colleague, blessed with high emotional intelligence, had intuitively read my mind. And it suddenly hit me that no one at work had ever asked me how I was doing. And actually meant it, beyond a simple greeting. For five years I'd been working hard to give the impression I was OK. And telling myself the same thing every day. But there were some times when I really wasn't OK. And I realised this was one of them. Something cracked way down inside and it was all I could do to hold back the tears.

'Maybe. But I really don't want to talk right now,' was all I could say. I didn't mean it rudely. My colleague nodded and didn't press for more. She politely left to give me some space. I went to a familiar hiding place, the men's toilets, where I stood in the corner of a cubicle and I cried. And when I'd finished crying I felt really, really good.

That's when I knew I'd done the right thing. After all of that stifled tension drained away, my energy quickly came back. And diverted itself to a new place.

I missed freelancing and knew I wanted to get back to that way of working. But maybe this time I could do something bigger. Maybe I could team up with other freelancers, set up a mini studio and go after some clients on my own. I was already in mid-career and it felt like a case of now or never. I put out the feelers and just as I left my position, in the first few days of 2020, I landed my first client. I was working on-site, in a much calmer office, with fewer company-wide demands on my plate. And it felt great. The work got extended into spring. It was looking like it would run through until summer.

But then the coronavirus arrived. And the whole world turned upside down.

Almost immediately, everyone was sent away to work from home. I'd often worked from home in the past, when there were problems with the trains or my kids got sick. Or when I just needed to get my head down for the day and really plough through some work. But now here we were, absolutely all of us, working remotely five days a week. People working together but never together.

It was a novelty at first but I understand why some people quickly started hating it. If you get your energy from the hustle and buzz of the office, being alone at home all day must feel like being cast adrift at sea. A loss of focus, a lack of momentum. I heard so many people describing remote working almost in terms of pain. *I can't stand it. It's killing me. When will it stop?* They didn't like the new normal and couldn't wait to get back to regular office life. In some ways COVID-19 has been like a personal litmus test. It quickly showed who needs to have people around them, inside and outside of work. And who doesn't.

Unsurprisingly, I've always been more productive when I work from home. Without the daily commute to worry about I can be showered, fed and at my computer by 8am. Without all the noise and the constant interruptions of an open plan office, I find a deeper level of focus. And get a hell of a lot more done. Before the workday is over I feel like I've achieved twice as much. I've heard people describing 'flow' before. When they're so absorbed in something they completely lose themselves and any awareness of the world around them. But their performance itself gets a significant boost. When they leave their flow state they'll find they've done their best work of the day. Output that's twice as good, in half the time.

I've never experienced flow like that in a crowded workspace.

In the office I used to look for places to run away to, so I could concentrate. I'd sit behind some fake bushes, bent low over my laptop. Sometimes I'd sit at the back of a cafe, desperately seeking some of that elusive flow. But when I'm at home, in my own space, with enough quiet, the flow comes to me. In the first few weeks and months of COVID-19, working in this way felt life-changing.

It goes without saying that the biggest benefit for me was a physical separation from people. Working remotely all day, every week, gave me a sense of control I'd never had before. The office wasn't dictating my day anymore. Yes, there were meetings in calendars and Zoom calls to join and deadlines we all had to hit. In terms of work my employers still drove my daily activity. But mentally and emotionally I was completely free of a communal social environment. All the things that habitually frightened me, like unexpected conversations or lots of people seeing me blush, were now gone. At home I can control all the variables and there are very few surprises.

Even the events that typically troubled me the most, like talking in groups or presenting to a client, have become much more manageable. I find it easier to speak to people through a computer screen. Being one step removed from them makes all the difference. When I'm talking to lots of people online, it's harder for them to see me blush. We're not in the same room and I don't feel trapped. I'm in less perceived danger and I relax more. When I'm presenting a document to a client I'm still nervous and self-conscious. That will never go away completely. But my face, my body, my whole physical existence has shrunk down to a little square in the corner of the screen. My voice stays centre-stage but my red skin does not. I've taken one step back from the spotlight. One step back from myself, even. It means I think better. I present better. I feel protected and my phobia runs out of steam.

In my old role I took too many beta blockers. I swallowed them every time I had an important meeting coming up. It was another sign that something had to change and my environment was getting the better of me. I've now stopped taking beta blockers altogether. There just aren't enough occasions when I need them anymore. You know that black zeppelin that drifts onto the horizon before a challenging social moment? It doesn't get off the ground much these days. Because all of these social encounters are being handled remotely, I'm fearing them a great deal less. The anticipation doesn't get a chance to grow. So the vicious cycle is slowing down. I can feel my SAD diminishing.

Please don't get me wrong: I know the immense damage COVID has wreaked on so many people. I can't begin to contemplate all the lives lost, the families broken, the jobs destroyed, the dreams crushed, on our own doorsteps and right across the world.

But for the first time in living memory, we've been exposed to a new way of living and working. Working from home suddenly became mandatory. But not so long ago 'WFH' was almost a dirty little euphemism. It meant slacking off while your boss couldn't see you, kicking back in the middle of the day to watch some daytime TV. But collectively we've shown as a workforce that it's not like that at all. People can be trusted to manage their own time and workload. And do it all unmonitored. A great deal of us even seem to thrive on this approach. Until now I'd accepted my whole career would be one long fight against social anxiety. And the battlefield would always be the workplace. But in the space of one year that whole idea has been flipped on its head.

The same goes for social settings outside of work. There are fewer of them now, and I feel my anxiety dropping notch by notch. This even applies to my own 40th birthday. I'd planned to throw a party, the venue had been booked and all the guests had been invited. I wanted to celebrate the big 4-0 like all my other friends had but inevitably I was worrying and fretting about it well in advance. About being the centre of attention and making it through the night without turning red. When we eventually cancelled the whole thing, a cool wave of relief washed right through me.

Which is why I also need to acknowledge there's another side to this coin. And it's a dangerous one to ignore. Social distancing has made life easier for me on many levels. But it might make life harder in the long run. Already I can feel my discomfort more keenly when I'm suddenly thrown back into direct human contact. The adrenaline flows fast, the blush comes quick. Dealing with social anxiety is like flexing a muscle and I can't delude myself that I don't need to keep on practising. It took me three decades to reach the point I'm at now. I worry it could all be undone in record time if I sit back and relax too much. Human contact, in the flesh, will always be important. Even for someone like me.

But big changes are coming. You can feel it. The truth is we will never return to work as we used to know it. Subconsciously, it's the kind of change I've always craved. Consciously, it's one I've grabbed with both hands.

The social distancing of COVID-19 has made life hard. But it's temporary. The social distance making its way into our professional lives looks like it will stick around a lot longer. In the right moderation, I'm absolutely certain it will make all of our lives better.

# 23. Why?

**W**hy did I write this book? It's a hard question to answer because so much of what I've said in here goes against my natural instincts. I don't like to talk about myself. It makes me feel awkward and self-indulgent. Self-worthy, even. As I've written these pages I've been hyper-conscious of all the I, I, I. The me, me, me. Everything I write in my professional life is anonymous: copywriters live in the third-person, their name is missing from their work, their words belong to somebody else. So writing about myself, as myself, opening up some very private thoughts that many people — including members of my own family — will be reading for the first time. Well, why do it? Why put myself in that position and talk out loud when nobody has asked to hear it?

I suppose it's because I've spent 40 years not talking about it. And everywhere you look, problems get worse if we hide them. As I approach middle age, the thought of going through the rest of life without ever talking about the fear that has dogged my every move since childhood would feel like a disavowal of myself, of anyone else who's ever lived with social anxiety. Almost by definition Social Anxiety Disorder is something that people won't (can't) step forward to talk about. It's not new, people have struggled with it for generations. But most of these people have gone through life quietly, covertly, trying their very hardest not to draw attention to themselves. They've internalised everything, feeling like something was wrong with them, taking the guilt to the grave. I don't want to do that. I'd rather talk about it, even if the talking is uncomfortable.

The public conversation about mental health is getting bigger. It's rapidly becoming the zeitgeist. But it's a huge subject and we still don't talk enough. Men certainly don't. Beyond the top layer of bravado spread thinly over male life, there is an ocean of unresolved conflict that most men never address. In 2021, two decades into the 21st century, talking about weakness still feels like an act of self-sabotage. So men instinctively won't do it. And our problems simply sit in the shadows, festering. If we don't talk how will anyone ever know what's really going on? How will we ever see the true picture? Or find the best ways forward to make life better?

There are many vicious cycles in this book. And they're not confined to the thought patterns of SAD. Society is cyclical too.

People who don't speak about their problems often have parents who didn't speak about their problems. And their own children will be less likely to speak about their problems, too.

People tell me I'm very British, very buttoned-up and self-reserved. I suppose it's true and that's how I come across, partly because of anxiety but also partly down to British culture. We aren't renowned for our openness: our national character is awkward, apologetic, restrained. This, too, perpetuates in cycles and it's helped to colour who I am. But I'm trying hard to be more open as a parent. To talk things through with my kids, not skirt around them because they're difficult to tackle or even personally embarrassing for me. My kids will inevitably be British too. But perhaps they'll be a little closer to their inner selves. And willing to share that inner world with others. At least I hope so.

One thing I think about a lot is inheritance. If the ingredients for social anxiety live inside me, have they been passed on to my children? Will they be more susceptible to blushing, will the blushing make them uncomfortable around other people? As they grow older and their social sphere becomes more complex, will they withdraw from that discomfort – and later start to fear it? This is a long process and takes years to develop; my SAD didn't truly arrive until my late teens. But having been through it, I know the warning signs I'll be watching for as my children come of age and enter their early twenties.

Both my son and my daughter have olive skin, almost Mediterranean-looking after they've spent a summer in the sunshine. But when they've been running around like lunatics, their faces turn crimson. Sometimes, when I come through the front gate at nursery to pick them up at the end of the day, I spot them easily in a blur of hyperactive children — because their faces are glowing the reddest. Bright beetroot cheeks, their foreheads and hair drenched in sweat. But they're just little kids, growing into themselves. Maybe I'm seeing something when there's nothing there to see. Or maybe some early seeds have been sown. Either way, it's my job to embrace it and teach them to embrace themselves. If they blush, I don't want blushing to become a stigma. Because that's what it so quickly becomes when people with social anxiety are left to figure it all out on their own.

This book has been my personal story of that stigma and I can only speak for myself. But there are times when I see the signs of SAD in other adults, too. The seeds in them have grown and branched out over time into their own web of coping systems. There is a woman I work with who blushes. She obviously hates it and uses her hair to hide her face when it happens. But she's also developed an interesting strategy of owning it. When she goes red, she calls attention to it before anyone else can. She'll say: *Look how red I've gone!* Or: *Oh my god could I be any redder?* It's an instinctive reaction, almost as automatic as the blush itself. What I notice in others when she does this is how little they actually care. They probably wouldn't have mentioned it if she hadn't, it's always a bigger deal for her than it is for them. Usually they're keen to move on and almost find it irritating that she's dwelling on it. I can tell it all bothers her a lot. But she gets my respect for facing her fear so directly.

At the other end of the scale, and it feels telling that this next example is a man, was a guy I worked with once who had vivid ginger hair, pale skin and a powerful case of blushing. He would turn very red very easily, just like me. And he'd developed lots of strategies to deflect attention from himself. One was male banter, the quick ability to project humiliation away from you and onto somebody else. He was a master at this, to the point that his humour had become cutting – almost cruel – in an effort to avoid his anxiety. If the setting was more professional, too serious for banter, and a blush was slowly rising up into his face, he'd developed the habit of transferring what he was saying over to other people. His sentences would become questions that only other people could finish: *Oh yeah, we can do that, but I think the files are all on that server...?* And he would look questioningly at the person who'd told him the files were on a server. He already knew where both the files and the server were, but by shifting the flow of talk to somebody else, he forced them to pick up the sentence where he'd left off.

He would be absent from his desk for long periods of time. During those hours, nobody knew where he was. On his last day in the office, towards the end of the afternoon, he was nowhere to be seen. Then, five minutes before he was due to pack up and go, he suddenly turned up and emptied out his desk in a flurry of activity — as though he'd been detained in a meeting somewhere else in the building and now had to rush through his goodbyes. Just like the office goodbyes I always used to hate, all that attention focused on you with absolutely nowhere to hide. Best to avoid it if you can with some careful decoy tactics. The tell-tale signs were all there. I don't know if anyone else could see them.

These were, no doubt, just a few of the personal tics he'd developed over time to preserve himself from SAD. What made matters worse was that, like a lot of men who have a problem they seemingly can't fix, he had a big problem with alcohol. It was his crutch and his coping mechanism and his response to a lifetime of navigating through social anxiety on his own. I felt very much on his side but at the same time I knew he was becoming his own worst enemy. Left unchecked, this invisible web he'd built around himself would define the rest of his life: heavy drinking, social avoidance, one long, drawn-out plan of escape.

At the extreme end of the scale, you'll find stories from people like a young American man named Brandon Thomas, who found his blushing so traumatising that he took his own life, to the shock and grief of his family and everyone who knew him, at the age of 20. His tragedy has so much resonance for me and for people trying to make sense of their social anxiety. For anyone who doesn't know what SAD is or how blushing can take control of a person's life, you don't need to read my book. You just need to read this single paragraph written by Brandon himself. He captured it better than I can:

*'I blush several times a day. It doesn't have to be when I am embarrassed either. Things like when I'm at a grocery store and I see someone I know. I might actually want to talk to them, but I also don't want to because I know I will blush in front of them. I sometimes blush even if they don't see me. I definitely blush if I actually do run into someone I know anywhere, when I am not expecting to run into them. I blush when called on in class, or when I speak up in class. I blush when the attention is on me, even when I am with a group of people I am very comfortable with. If for example, someone says 'Hey Brandon tell everyone that story you told me,' I will blush, even if I really want to tell the story. Blushing sometimes affects what I do in life. At school I sometimes don't use the elevator with fear that it will stop on another floor and someone I know gets on. I even blush*

*in the car sometimes even when I'm alone. If I make a mistake driving, I sometimes blush. At night, when I think about instances where I have blushed, sometimes I blush, or at least feel my face get warm. I am tired of blushing. It is exhausting to wake up every day and have to find little ways to avoid blushing.'*

Since Brandon's death, his parents have set up an online support group to raise awareness of chronic blushing. This was their son's final wish and the site created in his honour is full of testimonials from people looking for help, people expressing their thanks, people telling their own stories of Social Anxiety Disorder. And all of that became possible because his parents chose to talk, to share, to educate others to stop more tragedies in the future. That mission has inspired me. At the very least, I hope this book will help just one person who's at their wit's end, who feels like they're stuck on the outside of life and can't get back in, who's convinced that nothing will ever get better. The message I hope you take away from here is simply this: things will get better and you're not on your own.

The more that people understand SAD, the more solidarity they can give. I'm not just talking about your friends and family – although they should be the first to know and accept that you're not just a bit bashful, you're not just a bit quiet, you're not just going through a phase. When your loved ones become aware that everything they find so easy is so hard for you, the weight of social anxiety lifts a little. It's not your dirty little secret anymore, it's not your private burden to carry alone. You'll have people who know your difficulties and what you're going through. It's amazing what a difference it can make when your private fear is in the open.

But what about when you're at work, when you're with your boss and your colleagues and surrounded by people who might be less forgiving? It shouldn't be any different there. Most companies today encourage people to take the Myers-Briggs test, a simple questionnaire that indicates where your personality lands on the Introvert/Extrovert scale. The results can help managers and resourcing teams put the right people on the right projects. And get a more human profile of their workforce. But it shouldn't stop there, at a simplified psychological test. Diversity at work is a major topic and rightly so, from gender and ethnicity to age and sexual orientation. Companies are slowly waking up to a more diverse workplace, not least because of the legal implications they could face if they don't. But to be truly inclusive, employers need to extend even further, into the finer points of Neurodiversity – a concept that says the neurological differences between people should be recognised and respected just as much as any physical differences.

But therein lies the problem: you can't see the neurological differences between people on the outside. They aren't plainly visible like sex or race or age. They live within the human brain, on a spectrum. They vary from Autism, to Tourette's, to Attention Deficit Hyperactivity Disorder, to Dyslexia, to Dysnomia, to Obsessive Compulsive Disorder – and there's no reason why it shouldn't include Social Anxiety Disorder. The list is still growing.

Whatever the condition, some people find themselves high up the scale, others find themselves down low. But the distressing fact is this: most workplaces don't recognise there's a spectrum there at all. The stuff that goes on inside your head? The brain you were born with? Well, that's just beyond their control – and when you start using words like 'disorder', people start thinking 'mental illness' – and all kinds of biases, unconscious or otherwise, start creeping in. I don't think I'd ever feel comfortable going to an HR department and telling them I have a social disorder, having it officially added to my records, knowing that from that point onwards they'd always see me differently. It would feel like I'd owned up to something that was best kept a secret, or even worse – that people would quietly think I was making a big deal out of something that wasn't real. Like when someone says they're lactose intolerant and people joke behind their backs: *You mean you just don't like milk?* I'd worry that people might be thinking something similar about me. *You mean you just don't like public speaking? No one does. Join the club!*

I still firmly believe what I said at the start of this book: you cannot have a curse without a blessing. What's been labelled as a disorder is not a one-way ticket to a lower quality of life. You may feel like it's a curse but it's also a gift that can improve other areas of your life. Certain kinds of people are suited to certain things. If you're socially anxious then you're skilled at spending time alone, at finding deep creative or analytical flow. It's no accident that good writers tend to be quieter people who thrive on solitude. It's no accident that good coders tend to be introverts who work wearing headphones. Who you are is driven by your genes, the way you were wired at birth, but it also comes from what you do, what you practice. When you want to get away from other people, you're not giving in to a weakness — you're honing a skill. All the time, because you're just doing what you naturally do, you're getting better at something. Be it writing, painting, coding, calculating. The curse and the blessing are intertwined. And it gets to a point where the blessing gains the upper hand.

Every day I'm in an office, I still feel like I'm forcing my character to go against its grain. I'm never fully at ease, I'm always aware that something inside me is hesitating and doesn't feel at home. But that's the smaller part of who I am now. I worry about it now much less than before.

Because you should never have to worry about who you are. In groups, human beings are full of complex contradictions. You're one of us, you're not one of us, we understand you, we don't understand you. There are social codes, prejudices, pitfalls and barriers all around us – so often unseen and unspoken – steering the way things get done. It will take time and big cultural change but one day we'll be in a different place, living in a new kind of reality, where all shades of psychological grey have been interpreted. Professionally and privately, everyone will be represented, nobody will be swept to the side, social anxiety and 'the illness of missed opportunities' won't be a mark of shame anymore.

It will be the start of a new world of opportunities.

# Acknowledgements

I'm amazed this book has made it into your hands. All in all it took me three years to write. Mostly standing up on packed trains as they rattled in and out of London Waterloo. When I was tapping awkwardly on a tablet balanced in the crook of my arm, it felt like it would take me 10 years to complete. How would I ever get there, writing in 30-minute bursts before and after work?

Fortunately my publisher gave me some great advice early on. 'Don't get it right, just get it down.' It pushed me to keep on writing without looking back. And it's the only way I got to the finish line. So, many thanks goes to Martin Hickman at Canbury Press for this vital creative hack. And for all the insights and encouragement you gave along the way. Thanks for the editing expertise, when the writing really gets done. And thanks most of all for answering an unsolicited email three years ago, from a total stranger, asking if you might want to tell a story about social anxiety.

Thanks to Katharine Nelson at Canbury, for keeping a sharp eye on the marketing. And Ella Davidson and Emma Preece at The Book Publicist for driving all our PR.

Thanks to my mum and dad for answering all the questions I had about the early years. I told you I was writing a book about introverts. By now you know it's more than that. And you should both know you're more than parents. You're friends and guides and you've given me absolutely everything I've ever needed in life.

I owe a great deal to my wife, Deep. You agreed to appear in this book and gave me the space to make it happen. Whenever I was writing, you were parenting. Thank you for making so many sacrifices and supporting me all the way.

Thanks to my little boy and my little girl for your constant joy. Both of you make me a better person and each day better than the last.

Finally, thanks to all the people whose work and outlook on life made me feel a book like this was even possible in the first place. Susan Cain and her empowerment of introverts. Grayson Perry and his reboot of masculinity. The parents of Brandon Thomas, who set up *chronicblushinghelp.com* to raise awareness of uncontrollable blushing. If this kind of content wasn't out there in the world, gently making a difference, I probably wouldn't have written *Redface*.

We owe it to ourselves to keep speaking up about our mental health. I hope some of the things you've read in here might inspire you to say a little more, too.

Help with social anxiety is available

from the charity Anxiety UK

**Opening hours**

Monday to Friday: 9.30am – 5.30pm

**Helpline**

03444 775 774

**Website**

www.anxietyuk.org.uk

**Email (not instant response)**

support@anxietyuk.org.uk

**Text (not instant response)**

07537 416 905

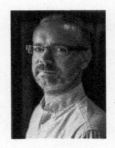

Russell Norris is a copywriter. After battling Social Anxiety Disorder for years, he became an executive at a leading advertising agency in London. He now runs his own business. He lives in south London with his family. This is his first non-fiction book.